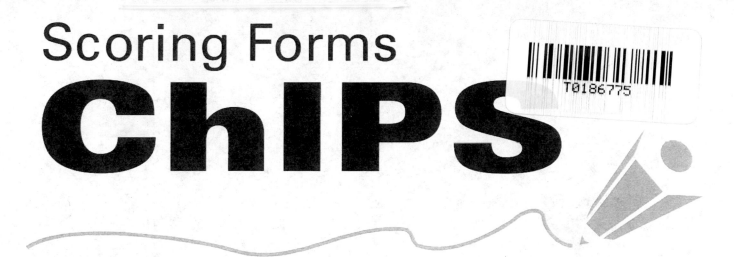

Scoring Forms
ChIPS

Also available from American Psychiatric Publishing Group (1-800-368-5777; www.appi.org)

■ **ChIPS—Children's Interview for Psychiatric Syndromes** (Item #8398)
(reusable interview administration booklet)

Based on strict DSM-IV criteria and validated in more than 12 years of studies, the ChIPS is brief and simple to administer. Questions are succinct, simply worded, and easily understood by children and adolescents. Practitioners in clinical and research settings alike have already found the ChIPS indispensable in screening for conditions such as attention-deficit/hyperactivity disorder, conduct disorder, substance abuse, phobias, anxiety disorders, stress disorders, eating disorders, mood disorders, elimination disorders, and schizophrenia.

Scoring Form for ChIPS, package of 20 (Item #8846)
(one-time-use booklet for recording answers, with Profile Sheet)

Scoring Forms provide ample space for recording verbatim responses to interview questions, with check boxes to indicate whether symptom criteria and duration and impairment requirements are met. A Profile Sheet, perforated for easy removal from the Scoring Form, is included to itemize principal findings and diagnoses.

Report Form for ChIPS, package of 20 (Item #8899)
(one-time-use abbreviated summary form)

Report Forms provide a quick way of conveying ChIPS results. If subsequently desired, this "at-a-glance" summary of the symptoms endorsed during the interview can be used by a clinician to identify areas warranting further scrutiny.

■ **P-ChIPS—Children's Interview for Psychiatric Syndromes—Parent Version** (Item #8847)
(reusable interview administration booklet)

The Parent Version of the ChIPS essentially consists of the same interview text altered from second to third person to address the parent rather than the child (e.g., "Have you ever" is changed to "Has your child ever").

Scoring Form for P-ChIPS, package of 20 (Item #8396)
(one-time-use booklet for recording answers, with Profile Sheet)

Report Form for P-ChIPS, package of 20 (Item #8399)
(one-time-use abbreviated summary form)

■ **Administration Manual** (Item #8849)

Covering both the ChIPS and the P-ChIPS, the Administration Manual is informative and user-friendly. It presents background information about the interview's development, detailed instructions for conducting the interview and recording its results, explicit criteria for assessing interviewee responses, complete specifications for preparing mental health paraprofessionals to administer the interview, and illustrative case studies.

ISBN 978-0-88048-846-4

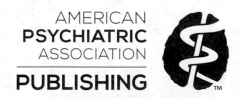

AMERICAN
PSYCHIATRIC
ASSOCIATION
PUBLISHING

ENU

Criteria
If 1, ≥1 in 2, 3a, and 3b,
then criteria met
ENU < >

Duration
1. _____ (years old)
2. < > _____ (years old)
3. <a> _____ (x/week)
   <b> _____ (months)
*DUR met for ENU < >

Impairment
1. < > home
2. < > school
3. < > peers

ENC

Type
Nocturnal < >
Diurnal < >
Both < >

1. < >
2. < >

Criteria
If both 1 & 2, then criteria met
ENC < >

Duration
1. _____ (years old)
2. < > _____ (years old)
3. <a> _____ (x/month)
   <b> _____ (months)
*DUR met for ENC < >

Impairment
1. < > home
2. < > school
3. < > peers

SCZ/PSY

A. Psychotic Symptoms
1. <a> <b> <c> <e>
2. <a> <b> <c> <d> <e> <f>
3. < >
4. < >
5. < >

B. Interference
1. < >
2. < >
3. < >

Criteria
If ≥2 in A and ≥1 in B,
then criteria met
SCZ < >
If ≥1 in A, then criteria met
PSY < >

Duration
1. _____ (years old)
2. < > _____ (years old)
3. < > _____ (months)
*DUR met for SCZ < >
*DUR met for PSY < >

STRESSORS

A. Child Abuse/Neglect
1. <a> <b> <c>
2. <a> <b> <c> <d>
3. <a> <b> <c> <d>
4. < >
5. < >

Duration
1. _____
2. < > _____
3. _____
4. _____
5. < > _____

B. Other Stressors
1. <a> <b> <c> <d> <e>
2. < >
3. <a> <b>
4. <a> <b> <c>
5. <a> <b>
6. <a> <b>
7. <a> _____
   <b> _____
8. <a> <b> <c> <d>
9. < > _____
10. < > _____
11. < > _____

DEP/DYS (MDD/DD)	DEP/DYS (MDD/DD)	MAN/HYPOMAN

A. Dysphoric Mood
  1. \<a\> \<b\> \<c\>
  2. \<a\> \<bi\> \<bii\> \<biii\>
     \<c\> \<d\>
 	
B. Loss of Interest
  1. \<a\> \<b\>
  2. \<a\> \<b\> \<c\>
 	
C. Appetite Changes
  1. \<a\> \<b\> \<c\>
  2. \<a\> \<b\>
 	
D. Sleep Changes
     Bedtime: _____
     Wakeup: _____
  1. \<a\> \<b\> \<c\>
  2. \<a\> \<b\>
 	
E. Psychomotor Changes
  1. \<a\> \<b\> \<c\> \<d\>
  2. \<a\> \<b\>
 	
F. Low Energy
  1. \<a\> \<b\> \<c\> \<d\>
 	
G. Guilt
  1. \<a\> \<b\> \<c\> \<d\>
  2. \<a\> \<b\>
 	
H. Impaired Concentration
  1. \<a\> \<b\> \<c\> \<d\> \<e\>
  2. \< \>
 	
I. Hopelessness
  1. \<a\> \<b\> \<c\>
 	
J. Morbid/Suicidal Thoughts
  1. \<a\> \<b\>
  2. \<a\> \<b\> \<c\> \<d\> \<e\>
 	
_____
_____
_____
_____
_____
		A. Elevated Mood
		  1. \<a\> _____
		     \<b\> _____
		     \<c\> _____
		  2. \< \> _____
		
		B. Other Symptoms
		  1. \<a\> _____
		     \<b\>
		  2. \<a\> \<b\> \<c\> _____
		  3. \<a\> \<b\> \<c\> \<d\>
		  4. \<a\> \<b\> \<c\>
		  5. \< \>
		  6. \<a\> \<b\> \<c\> \<d\> \<e\>
		  7. \<a\> \<b\> \<c\> \<d\>
		
		C. Interference
		  1. \< \>
		  2. \< \>

	Criteria
	  If A &/or B & ≥5 of A–H or J,
	    then criteria met
	    MDD \< \>
	
	  If A & ≥2 of C, D, F, G, H, or I,
	    then criteria met
	    DD \< \>
		Criteria
		  If A1(a, b, & c) + ≥3 in B + ≥1 in C
		    or
		  A2 + ≥4 in B + ≥1 in C,
		    then criteria met
		    MAN \< \>
		
		  If A1(a, b, & c) + ≥3 in B +
		    none in C
		    or
		  A2 + ≥4 in B + none in C,
		    then criteria met
		    HYPOMAN \< \>

	Duration
	  1. _____ (years old)
	  2. \< \> _____ (years old)
	  3. MDD \< \> _____ (weeks)
	    DD \< \> _____ (months)
	
	    *DUR met for MDD \< \>
	    *DUR met for DD \< \>
		Duration
		  1. _____ (years old)
		  2. \< \> _____ (years old)
		  3. MAN \< \> _____ (weeks)
		    HYPO \< \> _____ (days)
		
		    *DUR met for MAN \< \>
		    *DUR met for HYPOMAN \< \>

	Impairment
	  1. \< \> home
	  2. \< \> school
	  3. \< \> peers
		Impairment
		  1. \< \> home
		  2. \< \> school
		  3. \< \> peers

STRESS (ASD/PTSD)	ANO	BUL

A. Exposure
1. <a> <b>
2. <a> <b> <c> <d> <e>
3. < >
B. Dissociation
1. <a> <b> <c> <d>
2. < >
3. < >
4. < >
5. < >
C. Reexperiencing
1. <a> <b> <c>
2. <a> <b>
3. <a> <b>
4. <a> <b>
5. < >
D. Avoidance
1. <a> <b>
2. <a> <b> <c>
3. < >
4. <a> <b>
5. <a> <b>
6. <a> <b>
7. <a> <b>
E. Hyperarousal
1. <a> <b>
2. <a> <b>
3. < >
4. < >
5. < >
	1. <a> <b>
	2. <a>
	  ht: _____
	  wt: _____
	  <b>
	3. <a> <b> <c>
	4. <a> <b> <c>
	5. < >
		1. < > _____
		2. <a> <b> <c> <d>
		  ht: _____
		  wt: _____
		3. <a> <b> <c> <d>
		4. <a> <b>

Criteria If A1 & A2, ≥3 in B, ≥1 in C, ≥3 in D, and ≥2 in E, then criteria met ASD < > If A1 & A2, ≥1 in C, ≥3 in D, and ≥2 in E, then criteria met PTSD < >	**Criteria** If 1–4 (≤5 for pubescent girls), then criteria met ANO < >	**Criteria** If 1–4, then criteria met BUL < >

Duration
1. _____ (years old)
2. < > _____ (years old)
3. a. < > _____ (weeks)
  b. < > _____ (days)
  c. < > _____ (days)
4. < > _____ (months)
*DUR met for ASD < >
*DUR met for PTSD < >
	Duration
	1. _____ (years old)
	2. < > _____ (years old)
	3. < > _____ (months)
	*DUR met for ANO < >
		Duration
		1. _____ (years old)
		2. < > _____ (years old)
		3. a. < > _____ (#/week)
		  b. < > _____ (months)
		*DUR met for BUL < >

Type (PTSD) Acute < > Regular Onset < > Chronic < > Delayed Onset < > **Impairment** 1. < > home 2. < > school 3. < > peers	**Impairment** 1. < > home 2. < > school 3. < > peers	**Impairment** 1. < > home 2. < > school 3. < > peers

SEP ANX	GEN ANX	OCD

1. <a> <b>
 2. <a> <b>
 3. < >
 4. <a> <b>
 5. <a> <b>
 6. <a> <b>
 7. <a> <b>
 8. <a> <b>
	1. < > _____
	 _____
	 _____
	 _____
	 _____
	 2. <a> <b>
	 3. <a> <b> <c> <d> <e> <f>
		A. Compulsions
		   1. < > _____
		   2. <a> _____
		     <b>
		   3. < >
		
		 B. Obsessions
		   1. <a> _____
		     <b> _____
		     <c> _____
		   2. <a> <b> <c>
		   3. < >
		
		 C. Interference
		   1. <a> <b> <c>

Criteria If ≥3, then criteria met SEP ANX < >	**Criteria** If 1–3, then criteria met GEN ANX < >	**Criteria** If A1, A2, & C, then criteria met Compulsions < > If B1, B2, & C, then criteria met Obsessions < > If Compulsions + and/or Obsessions +, then criteria met OCD < >
Duration 1. _____ (years old) 2. < > _____ (years old) 3. < > _____ (weeks) *DUR met for SEP ANX < >	**Duration** 1. _____ (years old) 2. < > _____ (years old) 3. < > _____ (months) *DUR met for GEN ANX < >	**Duration** 1. _____ (years old) 2. < > _____ (years old) _____ (months) *DUR met for OCD < >
Impairment 1. < > home 2. < > school 3. < > peers	**Impairment** 1. < > home 2. < > school 3. < > peers	**Impairment** 1. < > home 2. < > school 3. < > peers

SUB AB	PHO	SOCIAL PHO

1. < >
   <a>_____
   <b>_____
   <c>_____
 	
 _____
 2. < > _____
 3. < > _____
 4. < > _____
	1. _____
	   _____
	   _____
	 2. <a> <b>
	 3. <a> <b>
	 4. <ai> <aii> <aiii> <aiv> <b>
	 5. <a> <b>
		1. <a> <b>
		 2. < >
		 3. <a> <b>
		 4. <ai> <aii> <aiii> <aiv> <b>
		 5. < >

Duration
 1. _____ (years old)
 2. < > _____ (years old)
   _____ (months)
 	
   * DUR met for SUB AB < >
	Criteria
	   If 1–4, then criteria met
	   PHO < >
		Criteria
		   If 1–4, then criteria met
		   SOCIAL PHO < >

	Duration
	 1. _____ (years old)
	 2. < > _____ (years old)
	 3. < > _____ (months)
	
	   * DUR met for PHO < >
		Duration
		 1. _____ (years old)
		 2. < > _____ (years old)
		 3. < > _____ (months)
		
		   *DUR met for SOCIAL PHO < >

Impairment 1. <a> <b> 2. < > 3. <a> <b> 4. < >	**Impairment** 1. < > home 2. < > school 3. < > peers	**Impairment** 1. < > home 2. < > school 3. < > peers

Criteria
   If any use (Q1–4) and any
   impairment (1–4), then criteria
   met SUB AB < >
 	
 Type(s) _____
 _____
 _____
 _____
	Type(s)
	 Animal < >
	 Natural Environment < >
	 Blood–Injection–Injury < >
	 Situational < >
	 Other _____ < >	

Child's Name: _____

Date: _____

ADHD

A. Inattention
1. <a> <b>
2. < >
3. <a> <b>
4. <a> <b> <c>
5. < >
6. < >
7. < >
8. <a> <b>
9. <a> <b>

B. Hyperactivity–Impulsivity
1. <a> <b>
2. <a> <b>
3. < >
4. <a> <b>
5. < >
6. <a> <b>
7. < >
8. <a> <b>
9. <a> <b> <c>

Criteria
If ≥6 in A only, then criteria met
Inattentive < >

If ≥6 in B only, then criteria met
Hyperactive–Impulsive < >

If ≥6 in A and ≥6 in B,
then criteria met
Combined < >

Duration
1. _____ (years old)
2. < > _____ (years old)
3. < > _____ (months)
* DUR met for ADHD < >

Impairment
1. < > home
2. < > school
3. < > peers

ODD

1. <a> <b>
2. <a> <b>
3. <a> <b> <c> <d>
4. < >
5. <a> <b>
6. < >
7. < >
8. < >

Criteria
If ≥4, then criteria met
ODD < >

Duration
1. _____ (years old)
2. < > _____ (years old)
3. < > _____ (months)
* DUR met for ODD < >

Impairment
1. < > home
2. < > school
3. < > peers

CD

1. < >
2. <a> <b>
3. < >
4. < >
5. < >
6. < >
7. <a> <b>
8. <a> <b>
9. < >
10. <a> <b>
11. < >
12. < >
13. < >
14. < >
15. <a> <b>

Criteria
If ≥3, then criteria met
CD < >

Duration
1. _____ (years old)
2. < > _____ (years old)
3. < > _____ (months)
* DUR met for CD < >

Impairment
1. < > home
2. < > school
3. < > peers

Type
Childhood Onset < >
Adolescent Onset < >
Mild < >
Moderate < >
Severe < >

Presenting Problem

Home

1.

2.

School

1.

2.

3.

4.

5.

Peers/Work

1.

2.

3.

4.

5.

Medication

Type:

Dosage:

Child's Number: _____ Date: _____

Child's Name: _____ Time Started: _____

Date of Birth: _____ Age: _____ Time Ended: _____

Race: _____ Sex: _____ Interviewer: _____

Setting (circle one):   Inpatient,   Outpatient,   School,   Other Research Setting: _____

	Disorder	Symptoms	Diagnosis	Duration	Clinician's Diagnosis
ADHD	Attention-Deficit/Hyperactivity Disorder	<>	<>	<>	Axis I
	Type: Inattentive, Hyperactive–Impulsive, Combined				
ODD	Oppositional Defiant Disorder	<>	<>	<>	
CD	Conduct Disorder	<>	<>	<>	
	Onset: Childhood, Adolescent				
	Severity: Mild, Moderate, Severe				
SUBAB	Substance Abuse	<>	<>	<>	
	Substance(s): _____				
PHO	Specific Phobia	<>	<>	<>	Axis II
	Type: _____				
SOCPHO	Social Phobia	<>	<>	<>	
SEPANX	Separation Anxiety Disorder	<>	<>	<>	Axis III
GENANX	General Anxiety Disorder	<>	<>	<>	
OCD	Obsessive-Compulsive Disorder	<>	<>	<>	
PTSD	Posttraumatic Stress Disorder	<>	<>	<>	Axis IV
	Type: Acute, Chronic				
	Onset: Regular, Delayed				
ASD	Acute Stress Disorder	<>	<>	<>	
ANO	Anorexia	<>	<>	<>	Axis V
BUL	Bulimia	<>	<>	<>	current:
DEP	Major Depressive Disorder	<>	<>	<>	past year:
DYS	Dysthymic Disorder	<>	<>	<>	
MAN	Mania	<>	<>	<>	
HYPOMAN	Hypomania	<>	<>	<>	
ENU	Enuresis	<>	<>	<>	
	Type: Nocturnal, Diurnal, Both				
ENC	Encopresis	<>	<>	<>	
SCZ	Schizophrenia	<>	<>	<>	
PSY	Psychosis	<>	<>	<>	

Psychosocial Stressors:

Other Stressors:

Behavioral Observations

Appearance: Affect:

Effort: Level of Activity:

Unusual Behaviors:

Child's Number: _____ Date: _____

Child's Name: _____ Time Started: _____

Date of Birth: _____ Age: _____ Time Ended: _____

Race: _____ Sex: _____ Interviewer: _____

Setting (circle one):   Inpatient,   Outpatient,   School,   Other Research Setting: _____

	Disorder	Symptoms	Diagnosis	Duration	Clinician's Diagnosis
ADHD	**Attention-Deficit/Hyperactivity Disorder**	<>	<>	<>	Axis I
	Type: Inattentive, Hyperactive–Impulsive, Combined				
ODD	**Oppositional Defiant Disorder**	<>	<>	<>	
CD	**Conduct Disorder**	<>	<>	<>	
	Onset: Childhood, Adolescent				
	Severity: Mild, Moderate, Severe				
SUBAB	**Substance Abuse**	<>	<>	<>	
	Substance(s): _____				
PHO	**Specific Phobia**	<>	<>	<>	Axis II
	Type: _____				
SOCPHO	**Social Phobia**	<>	<>	<>	
SEPANX	**Separation Anxiety Disorder**	<>	<>	<>	Axis III
GENANX	**General Anxiety Disorder**	<>	<>	<>	
OCD	**Obsessive-Compulsive Disorder**	<>	<>	<>	
PTSD	**Posttraumatic Stress Disorder**	<>	<>	<>	Axis IV
	Type: Acute, Chronic				
	Onset: Regular, Delayed				
ASD	**Acute Stress Disorder**	<>	<>	<>	
ANO	**Anorexia**	<>	<>	<>	Axis V
BUL	**Bulimia**	<>	<>	<>	current:
DEP	**Major Depressive Disorder**	<>	<>	<>	past year:
DYS	**Dysthymic Disorder**	<>	<>	<>	
MAN	**Mania**	<>	<>	<>	
HYPOMAN	**Hypomania**	<>	<>	<>	
ENU	**Enuresis**	<>	<>	<>	
	Type: Nocturnal, Diurnal, Both				
ENC	**Encopresis**	<>	<>	<>	
SCZ	**Schizophrenia**	<>	<>	<>	
PSY	**Psychosis**	<>	<>	<>	

Psychosocial Stressors:

Other Stressors:

Behavioral Observations

Appearance: Affect:

Effort: Level of Activity:

Unusual Behaviors:

Presenting Problem

Home

1.

2.

School

1.

2.

3.

4.

5.

Peers/Work

1.

2.

3.

4.

5.

Medication

Type:

Dosage:

Child's Name: _____

Date: _____

ADHD	ODD	CD

A. Inattention
  1. \<a> \<b>
  2. \< >
  3. \<a> \<b>
  4. \<a> \<b> \<c>
  5. \< >
  6. \< >
  7. \< >
  8. \<a> \<b>
  9. \<a> \<b>
 	
B. Hyperactivity–Impulsivity
  1. \<a> \<b>
  2. \<a> \<b>
  3. \< >
  4. \<a> \<b>
  5. \< >
  6. \<a> \<b>
  7. \< >
  8. \<a> \<b>
  9. \<a> \<b> \<c>
	1. \<a> \<b>
	2. \<a> \<b>
	3. \<a> \<b> \<c> \<d>
	4. \< >
	5. \<a> \<b>
	6. \< >
	7. \< >
	8. \< >
		1. \< >
		2. \<a> \<b>
		3. \< >
		4. \< >
		5. \< >
		6. \< >
		7. \<a> \<b>
		8. \<a> \<b>
		9. \< >
		10. \<a> \<b>
		11. \< >
		12. \< >
		13. \< >
		14. \< >
		15. \<a> \<b>

Criteria If ≥6 in *A only*, then criteria met Inattentive \< > If ≥6 in *B only*, then criteria met Hyperactive–Impulsive \< > If ≥6 in A *and* ≥6 in B, then criteria met Combined \< >	**Criteria** If ≥4, then criteria met ODD \< >	**Criteria** If ≥3, then criteria met CD \< >

Duration
1. _____ (years old)
2. \< > _____ (years old)
3. \< > _____ (months)
 	
  * DUR met for ADHD \< >
	Duration
	1. _____ (years old)
	2. \< > _____ (years old)
	3. \< > _____ (months)
	
	  * DUR met for ODD \< >
		Duration
		1. _____ (years old)
		2. \< > _____ (years old)
		3. \< > _____ (months)
		
		  * DUR met for CD \< >

Impairment 1. \< > home 2. \< > school 3. \< > peers	**Impairment** 1. \< > home 2. \< > school 3. \< > peers	**Impairment** 1. \< > home 2. \< > school 3. \< > peers
		Type Childhood Onset \< > Adolescent Onset \< > Mild \< > Moderate \< > Severe \< >

SUB AB	PHO	SOCIAL PHO

1. < >
    <a>_____
    <b>_____
    <c>_____
 	
    _____
2. < > _____
3. < > _____
4. < > _____
	1. _____
	    _____
	    _____
	2. <a> <b>
	3. <a> <b>
	4. <ai> <aii> <aiii> <aiv> <b>
	5. <a> <b>
		1. <a> <b>
		2. < >
		3. <a> <b>
		4. <ai> <aii> <aiii> <aiv> <b>
		5. < >

Duration
1. _____ (years old)
2. < > _____ (years old)
    _____ (months)
 	
  * DUR met for SUB AB < >
	Criteria
	  If 1–4, then criteria met
	      PHO < >
		Criteria
		  If 1–4, then criteria met
		    SOCIAL PHO < >

	Duration
	1. _____ (years old)
	2. < > _____ (years old)
	3. < > _____ (months)
	
	  * DUR met for PHO < >
		Duration
		1. _____ (years old)
		2. < > _____ (years old)
		3. < > _____ (months)
		
		  *DUR met for SOCIAL PHO < >

Impairment 1. <a> <b> 2. < > 3. <a> <b> 4. < >	**Impairment** 1. < > home 2. < > school 3. < > peers	**Impairment** 1. < > home 2. < > school 3. < > peers

Criteria
  If any use (Q1–4) and any
  impairment (1–4), then criteria
    met SUB AB < >
 	
Type(s) _____
_____
_____
_____
	Type(s)
	Animal < >
	Natural Environment < >
	Blood–Injection–Injury < >
	Situational < >
	Other _____ < >	

SEP ANX	GEN ANX	OCD

1. <a> <b>
2. <a> <b>
3. < >
4. <a> <b>
5. <a> <b>
6. <a> <b>
7. <a> <b>
8. <a> <b>
	1. < > _____
	_____
	_____
	_____
	_____
	2. <a> <b>
	3. <a> <b> <c> <d> <e> <f>
		A. Compulsions
		  1. < > _____
		  2. <a> _____
		    <b>
		  3. < >
		
		B. Obsessions
		  1. <a> _____
		    <b> _____
		    <c> _____
		  2. <a> <b> <c>
		  3. < >
		
		C. Interference
		  1. <a> <b> <c>

Criteria If ≥3, then criteria met SEP ANX < >	**Criteria** If 1–3, then criteria met GEN ANX < >	**Criteria** If A1, A2, & C, then criteria met Compulsions < > If B1, B2, & C, then criteria met Obsessions < > If Compulsions + and/or Obsessions +, then criteria met OCD < >

Duration
1. _____ (years old)
2. < > _____ (years old)
3. < > _____ (weeks)
 	
  *DUR met for SEP ANX < >
	Duration
	1. _____ (years old)
	2. < > _____ (years old)
	3. < > _____ (months)
	
	  *DUR met for GEN ANX < >
		Duration
		1. _____ (years old)
		2. < > _____ (years old)
		_____ (months)
		
		  *DUR met for OCD < >

Impairment 1. < > home 2. < > school 3. < > peers	**Impairment** 1. < > home 2. < > school 3. < > peers	**Impairment** 1. < > home 2. < > school 3. < > peers

STRESS (ASD/PTSD)	ANO	BUL

A. Exposure
   1. \<a> \<b> _____
   2. \<a> \<b> \<c> \<d> \<e>
   3. \< > _____
B. Dissociation
   1. \<a> \<b> \<c> \<d>
   2. \< >
   3. \< >
   4. \< >
   5. \< >
C. Reexperiencing
   1. \<a> \<b> \<c>
   2. \<a> \<b>
   3. \<a> \<b>
   4. \<a> \<b>
   5. \< >
D. Avoidance
   1. \<a> \<b>
   2. \<a> \<b> \<c>
   3. \< >
   4. \<a> \<b>
   5. \<a> \<b>
   6. \<a> \<b>
   7. \<a> \<b>
E. Hyperarousal
   1. \<a> \<b>
   2. \<a> \<b>
   3. \< >
   4. \< >
   5. \< >
	1. \<a> \<b>
	2. \<a>
	   ht: _____
	   wt: _____
	  \<b>
	   ht: _____
	   wt: _____
	3. \<a> \<b> \<c>
	4. \<a> \<b> \<c>
	5. \< >
		1. \< > _____
		_____
		
		2. \<a> \<b> \<c> \<d>
		3. \<a> \<b> \<c> \<d>
		4. \<a> \<b>

Criteria If A1 & A2, ≥3 in B, ≥1 in C, ≥3 in D, and ≥2 in E, then criteria met ASD \< > If A1 & A2, ≥1 in C, ≥3 in D, and ≥2 in E, then criteria met PTSD \< >	**Criteria** If 1–4 (&5 for pubescent girls), then criteria met ANO \< >	**Criteria** If 1–4, then criteria met BUL \< >

Duration
1. _____ (years old)
2. \< > _____ (years old)
3. a. \< > _____ (weeks)
   b. \< >
   c. \< > _____ (days)
4. \< > _____ (months)
   *DUR met for ASD \< >
   *DUR met for PTSD \< >
	Duration
	1. _____ (years old)
	2. \< > _____ (years old)
	3. \< > _____ (months)
	
	   *DUR met for ANO \< >
		Duration
		1. _____ (years old)
		2. \< > _____ (years old)
		3. a. \< > _____ (#/week)
		   b. \< > _____ (months)
		
		   *DUR met for BUL \< >

Impairment 1. \< > home 2. \< > school 3. \< > peers	**Impairment** 1. \< > home 2. \< > school 3. \< > peers	**Impairment** 1. \< > home 2. \< > school 3. \< > peers
Type (PTSD) Acute \< > Regular Onset \< > Chronic \< > Delayed Onset \< >		

DEP/DYS (MDD/DD)	DEP/DYS (MDD/DD)	MAN/HYPOMAN

A. Dysphoric Mood
  1. \<a> \<b> \<c>
  2. \<a> \<bi> \<bii> \<biii>
    \<c> \<d>
 	
B. Loss of Interest
  1. \<a> \<b>
  2. \<a> \<b> \<c>
 	
C. Appetite Changes
  1. \<a> \<b> \<c>
  2. \<a> \<b>
 	
D. Sleep Changes
    Bedtime: _____
    Wakeup: _____
  1. \<a> \<b> \<c>
  2. \<a> \<b>
 	
E. Psychomotor Changes
  1. \<a> \<b> \<c> \<d>
  2. \<a> \<b>
 	
F. Low Energy
  1. \<a> \<b> \<c> \<d>
 	
G. Guilt
  1. \<a> \<b> \<c> \<d>
  2. \<a> \<b>
 	
H. Impaired Concentration
  1. \<a> \<b> \<c> \<d> \<e>
  2. \< >
 	
I. Hopelessness
  1. \<a> \<b> \<c>
 	
J. Morbid/Suicidal Thoughts
  1. \<a> \<b>
  2. \<a> \<b> \<c> \<d> \<e>
 	
_____
_____
_____
_____
_____
		A. Elevated Mood
		  1. \<a> _____
		    \<b> _____
		    \<c> _____
		  2. \< > _____
		
		B. Other Symptoms
		  1. \<a> _____
		    \<b>
		  2. \<a> \<b> \<c> _____
		  3. \<a> \<b> \<c> \<d>
		  4. \<a> \<b> \<c>
		  5. \< >
		  6. \<a> \<b> \<c> \<d> \<e>
		  7. \<a> \<b> \<c> \<d>
		
		C. Interference
		  1. \< >
		  2. \< >

	Criteria If A &/or B & ≥5 of A–H or J, then criteria met MDD \< > If A & ≥2 of C, D, F, G, H, or I, then criteria met DD \< >	**Criteria** If A1(a, b, & c) + ≥3 in B + ≥1 in C *or* A2 + ≥4 in B + ≥1 in C, then criteria met MAN \< > If A1(a, b, & c) + ≥3 in B + none in C *or* A2 + ≥4 in B + none in C, then criteria met HYPOMAN \< >

	Duration
	1. _____ (years old)
	2. \< > _____ (years old)
	3. MDD \< > _____ (weeks)
	    DD \< > _____ (months)
	
	  *DUR met for MDD \< >
	  *DUR met for DD \< >
		Duration
		1. _____ (years old)
		2. \< > _____ (years old)
		3. MAN \< > _____ (weeks)
		    HYPO \< > _____ (days)
		
		  *DUR met for MAN \< >
		  *DUR met for HYPOMAN \< >

	Impairment 1. \< > home 2. \< > school 3. \< > peers	**Impairment** 1. \< > home 2. \< > school 3. \< > peers

ENU	SCZ/PSY	STRESSORS

1. < >
2. <a> <b>
3. <a> <b>
	A. Psychotic Symptoms
	   1. <a> <b> <c> <d> <e>
	   2. <a> <b> <c> <d> <e> <f>
	   3. < >
	   4. < >
	   5. < >
		A. Child Abuse/Neglect
		   1. <a> <b> <c>
		   2. <a> <b> <c> <d>
		   3. <a> <b> <c> <d>
		   4. < >
		   5. < >

Criteria
  If 1, ≥1 in 2, 3a, and 3b,
    then criteria met
      ENU < >
	B. Interference
	   1. < >
	   2. < >
	   3. < >
		Duration
		1. _____
		2. < > _____
		3. _____
		4. _____
		5. < >

Duration
1. _____ (years old)
2. < > _____ (years old)
3. <a> _____ (x/week)
   <b> _____ (months)
 	
  *DUR met for ENU < >
	Criteria
	  If ≥2 in A and ≥1 in B,
	    then criteria met
	      SCZ < >
	
	  If ≥1 in A, then criteria met
	      PSY < >
		B. Other Stressors
		  1. <a> <b> <c> <d> <e>
		  2. < >
		  3. <a> <b>
		  4. <a> <b> <c>
		  5. <a> <b>
		  6. <a> <b>
		  7. <a> _____
		      <b>
		  8. <a> <b> <c> <d>
		  9. < > _____

Impairment
1. < > home
2. < > school
3. < > peers
	Duration
	1. _____ (years old)
	2. < > _____ (years old)
	3. < > _____ (months)
	
	  *DUR met for SCZ < >
	  *DUR met for PSY < >
		_____
		10. < > _____
		11. < > _____
		
		      _____
		      _____

Type Nocturnal < > Diurnal < > Both < >		
ENC	**Impairment** 1. < > home 2. < > school 3. < > peers	
1. < > 2. < >		
Criteria If both 1 & 2, then criteria met ENC < >		
Duration 1. _____ (years old) 2. < > _____ (years old) 3. <a> _____ (x/month) <b> _____ (months) *DUR met for ENC < >		
Impairment 1. < > home 2. < > school 3. < > peers		

ChIPS Scoring Form
Profile Sheet

Child's Number: _____ Date: _____

Child's Name: _____ Time Started: _____

Date of Birth: _____ Age: _____ Time Ended: _____

Race: _____ Sex: _____ Interviewer: _____

Setting (circle one): Inpatient, Outpatient, School, Other Research Setting: _____

	Disorder	Symptoms	Diagnosis	Duration	Clinician's Diagnosis
ADHD	**Attention-Deficit/Hyperactivity Disorder** *Type:* Inattentive, Hyperactive–Impulsive, Combined	<>	<>	<>	**Axis I**
ODD	**Oppositional Defiant Disorder**	<>	<>	<>	
CD	**Conduct Disorder** *Onset:* Childhood, Adolescent *Severity:* Mild, Moderate, Severe	<>	<>	<>	
SUBAB	**Substance Abuse** *Substance(s):* _____	<>	<>	<>	
PHO	**Specific Phobia** *Type:* _____	<>	<>	<>	**Axis II**
SOCPHO	**Social Phobia**	<>	<>	<>	
SEPANX	**Separation Anxiety Disorder**	<>	<>	<>	**Axis III**
GENANX	**General Anxiety Disorder**	<>	<>	<>	
OCD	**Obsessive-Compulsive Disorder**	<>	<>	<>	
PTSD	**Posttraumatic Stress Disorder** *Type:* Acute, Chronic *Onset:* Regular, Delayed	<>	<>	<>	**Axis IV**
ASD	**Acute Stress Disorder**	<>	<>	<>	
ANO	**Anorexia**	<>	<>	<>	**Axis V** current:
BUL	**Bulimia**	<>	<>	<>	past year:
DEP	**Major Depressive Disorder**	<>	<>	<>	
DYS	**Dysthymic Disorder**	<>	<>	<>	
MAN	**Mania**	<>	<>	<>	
HYPOMAN	**Hypomania**	<>	<>	<>	
ENU	**Enuresis** *Type:* Nocturnal, Diurnal, Both	<>	<>	<>	
ENC	**Encopresis**	<>	<>	<>	
SCZ	**Schizophrenia**	<>	<>	<>	
PSY	**Psychosis**	<>	<>	<>	

Psychosocial Stressors:

Other Stressors:

Behavioral Observations

Appearance: Affect:

Effort: Level of Activity:

Unusual Behaviors:

Presenting Problem

Home

1.

2.

School

1.

2.

3.

4.

5.

Peers/Work

1.

2.

3.

4.

5.

Medication

Type:

Dosage:

ADHD	ODD	CD

A. Inattention
  1. <a> <b>
  2. < >
  3. <a> <b>
  4. <a> <b> <c>
  5. < >
  6. < >
  7. < >
  8. <a> <b>
  9. <a> <b>
 	
B. Hyperactivity–Impulsivity
  1. <a> <b>
  2. <a> <b>
  3. < >
  4. <a> <b>
  5. < >
  6. <a> <b>
  7. < >
  8. <a> <b>
  9. <a> <b> <c>
	1. <a> <b>
	2. <a> <b>
	3. <a> <b> <c> <d>
	4. < >
	5. <a> <b>
	6. < >
	7. < >
	8. < >
		1. < >
		2. <a> <b>
		3. < >
		4. < >
		5. < >
		6. < >
		7. <a> <b>
		8. <a> <b>
		9. < >
		10. <a> <b>
		11. < >
		12. < >
		13. < >
		14. < >
		15. <a> <b>

Criteria If ≥6 in *A only*, then criteria met Inattentive < > If ≥6 in *B only*, then criteria met Hyperactive–Impulsive < > If ≥6 in A *and* ≥6 in B, then criteria met Combined < >	**Criteria** If ≥4, then criteria met ODD < >	**Criteria** If ≥3, then criteria met CD < >

Duration
1. _____ (years old)
2. < > _____ (years old)
3. < > _____ (months)
 	
  * DUR met for ADHD < >
	Duration
	1. _____ (years old)
	2. < > _____ (years old)
	3. < > _____ (months)
	
	  * DUR met for ODD < >
		Duration
		1. _____ (years old)
		2. < > _____ (years old)
		3. < > _____ (months)
		
		  * DUR met for CD < >

Impairment 1. < > home 2. < > school 3. < > peers	**Impairment** 1. < > home 2. < > school 3. < > peers	**Impairment** 1. < > home 2. < > school 3. < > peers
		Type Childhood Onset < > Adolescent Onset < > Mild < > Moderate < > Severe < >

SUB AB	PHO	SOCIAL PHO

1. < >
     <a>_____
     <b>_____
     <c>_____
 	
   _____
2. < > _____
3. < > _____
4. < > _____
	1. _____
	   _____
	   _____
	2. <a> <b>
	3. <a> <b>
	4. <ai> <aii> <aiii> <aiv> <b>
	5. <a> <b>
		1. <a> <b>
		2. < >
		3. <a> <b>
		4. <ai> <aii> <aiii> <aiv> <b>
		5. < >

Duration
1. _____ (years old)
2. < > _____ (years old)
    _____ (months)
 	
  * DUR met for SUB AB < >
	Criteria
	  If 1–4, then criteria met
	     PHO < >
		Criteria
		  If 1–4, then criteria met
		    SOCIAL PHO < >

	Duration
	1. _____ (years old)
	2. < > _____ (years old)
	3. < > _____ (months)
	
	   * DUR met for PHO < >
		Duration
		1. _____ (years old)
		2. < > _____ (years old)
		3. < > _____ (months)
		
		  *DUR met for SOCIAL PHO < >

Impairment 1. <a> <b> 2. < > 3. <a> <b> 4. < >	**Impairment** 1. < > home 2. < > school 3. < > peers	**Impairment** 1. < > home 2. < > school 3. < > peers

Criteria
  If any use (Q1–4) and any
  impairment (1–4), then criteria
    met SUB AB < >
 	
Type(s) _____
_____
_____
_____
	Type(s)
	Animal < >
	Natural Environment < >
	Blood–Injection–Injury < >
	Situational < >
	Other _____ < >	

SEP ANX	GEN ANX	OCD

1. \<a> \<b>
2. \<a> \<b>
3. \< >
4. \<a> \<b>
5. \<a> \<b>
6. \<a> \<b>
7. \<a> \<b>
8. \<a> \<b>
	1. \< > _____
	_____
	_____
	_____
	_____
	2. \<a> \<b>
	3. \<a> \<b> \<c> \<d> \<e> \<f>
		A. Compulsions
		  1. \< > _____
		  2. \<a> _____
		     \<b>
		  3. \< >
		
		B. Obsessions
		  1. \<a> _____
		     \<b> _____
		     \<c> _____
		  2. \<a> \<b> \<c>
		  3. \< >
		
		C. Interference
		  1. \<a> \<b> \<c>

Criteria
 	
   If ≥3, then criteria met
       SEP ANX \< >
	Criteria
	
	   If 1–3, then criteria met
	       GEN ANX \< >
		Criteria
		    If A1, A2, & C,
		   then criteria met
		   Compulsions \< >
		
		    If B1, B2, & C,
		   then criteria met
		   Obsessions \< >
		
		  If Compulsions +
		 and/or Obsessions +,
		   then criteria met
		     OCD \< >

Duration 1. _____ (years old) 2. \< > _____ (years old) 3. \< > _____ (weeks) *DUR met for SEP ANX \< >	**Duration** 1. _____ (years old) 2. \< > _____ (years old) 3. \< > _____ (months) *DUR met for GEN ANX \< >	**Duration** 1. _____ (years old) 2. \< > _____ (years old) _____ (months) *DUR met for OCD \< >
Impairment 1. \< > home 2. \< > school 3. \< > peers	**Impairment** 1. \< > home 2. \< > school 3. \< > peers	**Impairment** 1. \< > home 2. \< > school 3. \< > peers

STRESS (ASD/PTSD)	ANO	BUL

A. Exposure
  1. \<a> \<b> _____
  2. \<a> \<b> \<c> \<d> \<e>
  3. \< > _____
B. Dissociation
  1. \<a> \<b> \<c> \<d>
  2. \< >
  3. \< >
  4. \< >
  5. \< >
C. Reexperiencing
  1. \<a> \<b> \<c>
  2. \<a> \<b>
  3. \<a> \<b>
  4. \<a> \<b>
  5. \< >
D. Avoidance
  1. \<a> \<b>
  2. \<a> \<b> \<c>
  3. \< >
  4. \<a> \<b>
  5. \<a> \<b>
  6. \<a> \<b>
  7. \<a> \<b>
E. Hyperarousal
  1. \<a> \<b>
  2. \<a> \<b>
  3. \< >
  4. \< >
  5. \< >
	1. \<a> \<b>
	2. \<a>
	  ht: _____
	  wt: _____
	  \<b>
	  ht: _____
	  wt: _____
	3. \<a> \<b> \<c>
	4. \<a> \<b> \<c>
	5. \< >
		1. \< > _____
		  _____
		  _
		2. \<a> \<b> \<c> \<d>
		3. \<a> \<b> \<c> \<d>
		4. \<a> \<b>

Criteria If A1 *&* A2, ≥3 in B, ≥1 in C, ≥3 in D, and ≥2 in E, then criteria met ASD \< > If A1 *&* A2, ≥1 in C, ≥3 in D, and ≥2 in E, then criteria met PTSD \< >	**Criteria** If 1–4 (*&*5 for pubescent girls), then criteria met ANO \< >	**Criteria** If 1–4, then criteria met BUL \< >

Duration
1. _____ (years old)
2. \< > _____ (years old)
3. a. \< > _____ (weeks)
   b. \< >
   c. \< > _____ (days)
4. \< > _____ (months)
   *DUR met for ASD \< >
   *DUR met for PTSD \< >
	Duration
	1. _____ (years old)
	2. \< > _____ (years old)
	3. \< > _____ (months)
	
	   *DUR met for ANO \< >
		Duration
		1. _____ (years old)
		2. \< > _____ (years old)
		3. a. \< > _____ (#/week)
		   b. \< > _____ (months)
		
		   *DUR met for BUL \< >

Impairment 1. \< > home 2. \< > school 3. \< > peers	**Impairment** 1. \< > home 2. \< > school 3. \< > peers	**Impairment** 1. \< > home 2. \< > school 3. \< > peers
Type (PTSD) Acute \< > Regular Onset \< > Chronic \< > Delayed Onset \< >		

DEP/DYS (MDD/DD)	DEP/DYS (MDD/DD)	MAN/HYPOMAN
A. Dysphoric Mood 　1. \<a\> \<b\> \<c\> 　2. \<a\> \<bi\> \<bii\> \<biii\> 　　\<c\> \<d\> B. Loss of Interest 　1. \<a\> \<b\> 　2. \<a\> \<b\> \<c\> C. Appetite Changes 　1. \<a\> \<b\> \<c\> 　2. \<a\> \<b\> D. Sleep Changes 　　Bedtime: _____ 　　Wakeup: _____ 　1. \<a\> \<b\> \<c\> 　2. \<a\> \<b\> E. Psychomotor Changes 　1. \<a\> \<b\> \<c\> \<d\> 　2. \<a\> \<b\> F. Low Energy 　1. \<a\> \<b\> \<c\> \<d\> G. Guilt 　1. \<a\> \<b\> \<c\> \<d\> 　2. \<a\> \<b\> H. Impaired Concentration 　1. \<a\> \<b\> \<c\> \<d\> \<e\> 　2. \< \> I. Hopelessness 　1. \<a\> \<b\> \<c\> J. Morbid/Suicidal Thoughts 　1. \<a\> \<b\> 　2. \<a\> \<b\> \<c\> \<d\> \<e\> _____ _____ _____ _____ _____		A. Elevated Mood 　1. \<a\> _____ 　　\<b\> _____ 　　\<c\> _____ 　2. \< \> _____ B. Other Symptoms 　1. \<a\> _____ 　　\<b\> 　2. \<a\> \<b\> \<c\> _____ 　3. \<a\> \<b\> \<c\> \<d\> 　4. \<a\> \<b\> \<c\> 　5. \< \> 　6. \<a\> \<b\> \<c\> \<d\> \<e\> 　7. \<a\> \<b\> \<c\> \<d\> C. Interference 　1. \< \> 　2. \< \>
	Criteria If A &/or B & ≥5 of A–H or J, then criteria met MDD \< \> If A & ≥2 of C, D, F, G, H, or I, then criteria met DD \< \>	**Criteria** If A1(a, b, & c) + ≥3 in B + ≥1 in C *or* A2 + ≥4 in B + ≥1 in C, then criteria met MAN \< \> If A1(a, b, & c) + ≥3 in B + none in C *or* A2 + ≥4 in B + none in C, then criteria met HYPOMAN \< \>
	Duration 1. _____ (years old) 2. \< \> _____ (years old) 3. MDD \< \> _____ (weeks) 　DD \< \> _____ (months) 　*DUR met for MDD \< \> 　*DUR met for DD \< \>	**Duration** 1. _____ (years old) 2. \< \> _____ (years old) 3. MAN \< \> _____ (weeks) 　HYPO \< \> _____ (days) 　*DUR met for MAN \< \> 　*DUR met for HYPOMAN \< \>
	Impairment 1. \< \> home 2. \< \> school 3. \< \> peers	**Impairment** 1. \< \> home 2. \< \> school 3. \< \> peers

ENU	SCZ/PSY	STRESSORS

1. < >
2. \<a> \<b>
3. \<a> \<b>
	A. Psychotic Symptoms
	  1. \<a> \<b> \<c> \<d> \<e>
	  2. \<a> \<b> \<c> \<d> \<e> \<f>
	  3. < >
	  4. < >
	  5. < >
		A. Child Abuse/Neglect
		  1. \<a> \<b> \<c>
		  2. \<a> \<b> \<c> \<d>
		  3. \<a> \<b> \<c> \<d>
		  4. < >
		  5. < >

Criteria
    If 1, ≥1 in 2, 3a, and 3b,
      then criteria met
          ENU < >
	B. Interference
	  1. < >
	  2. < >
	  3. < >
		Duration
		  1. _____
		  2. < > _____
		  3. _____
		  4. _____
		  5. < >

Duration
  1. _____ (years old)
  2. < > _____ (years old)
  3. \<a> _____ (x/week)
     \<b> _____ (months)
 	
    *DUR met for ENU < >
	Criteria
	    If ≥2 in A and ≥1 in B,
	      then criteria met
	          SCZ < >
	
	    If ≥1 in A, then criteria met
	          PSY < >
		B. Other Stressors
		  1. \<a> \<b> \<c> \<d> \<e>
		  2. < >
		  3. \<a> \<b>
		  4. \<a> \<b> \<c>
		  5. \<a> \<b>
		  6. \<a> \<b>
		  7. \<a> _____
		       \<b>

Impairment
  1. < > home
  2. < > school
  3. < > peers
	Duration
	  1. _____ (years old)
	  2. < > _____ (years old)
	  3. < > _____ (months)
	
	    *DUR met for SCZ < >
	    *DUR met for PSY < >
		8. \<a> \<b> \<c> \<d>
		  9. < > _____
		       _____
		       _____
		  10. < >
		  11. < > _____
		       _____
		       _____

Type
Nocturnal   < >
Diurnal   < >
Both   < >
	Impairment
	  1. < > home
	  2. < > school
	  3. < > peers	

ENC		
1. < > 2. < >		
Criteria If both 1 & 2, then criteria met ENC < >		

Duration
  1. _____ (years old)
  2. < > _____ (years old)
  3. \<a> _____ (x/month)
     \<b> _____ (months)
 	
    *DUR met for ENC < >		

Impairment
  1. < > home
  2. < > school
  3. < > peers		

        ChIPS Scoring Form

ChIPS Scoring Form
Profile Sheet

Child's Number: _____   Date: _____

Child's Name: _____   Time Started: _____

Date of Birth: _____ Age: _____   Time Ended: _____

Race: _____ Sex: _____   Interviewer: _____

Setting (circle one):   Inpatient,   Outpatient,   School,   Other Research Setting: _____

	Disorder	Symptoms	Diagnosis	Duration	Clinician's Diagnosis
ADHD	**Attention-Deficit/Hyperactivity Disorder**	<>	<>	<>	Axis I
	Type: Inattentive, Hyperactive–Impulsive, Combined				
ODD	**Oppositional Defiant Disorder**	<>	<>	<>	
CD	**Conduct Disorder**	<>	<>	<>	
	Onset: Childhood, Adolescent				
	Severity: Mild, Moderate, Severe				
SUBAB	**Substance Abuse**	<>	<>	<>	
	Substance(s): _____				
PHO	**Specific Phobia**	<>	<>	<>	Axis II
	Type: _____				
SOCPHO	**Social Phobia**	<>	<>	<>	
SEPANX	**Separation Anxiety Disorder**	<>	<>	<>	Axis III
GENANX	**General Anxiety Disorder**	<>	<>	<>	
OCD	**Obsessive-Compulsive Disorder**	<>	<>	<>	
PTSD	**Posttraumatic Stress Disorder**	<>	<>	<>	Axis IV
	Type: Acute, Chronic				
	Onset: Regular, Delayed				
ASD	**Acute Stress Disorder**	<>	<>	<>	
ANO	**Anorexia**	<>	<>	<>	Axis V
BUL	**Bulimia**	<>	<>	<>	current:
DEP	**Major Depressive Disorder**	<>	<>	<>	past year:
DYS	**Dysthymic Disorder**	<>	<>	<>	
MAN	**Mania**	<>	<>	<>	
HYPOMAN	**Hypomania**	<>	<>	<>	
ENU	**Enuresis**	<>	<>	<>	
	Type: Nocturnal, Diurnal, Both				
ENC	**Encopresis**	<>	<>	<>	
SCZ	**Schizophrenia**	<>	<>	<>	
PSY	**Psychosis**	<>	<>	<>	

Psychosocial Stressors:

Other Stressors:

Behavioral Observations

Appearance: Affect:

Effort: Level of Activity:

Unusual Behaviors:

Presenting Problem

Home

1.

2.

School

1.

2.

3.

4.

5.

Peers/Work

1.

2.

3.

4.

5.

Medication

Type:

Dosage:

ChIPS Scoring Form

Child's Name: _____

Date: _____

ADHD	ODD	CD

A. Inattention
  1. \<a\> \<b\>
  2. \< \>
  3. \<a\> \<b\>
  4. \<a\> \<b\> \<c\>
  5. \< \>
  6. \< \>
  7. \< \>
  8. \<a\> \<b\>
  9. \<a\> \<b\>
 	
B. Hyperactivity–Impulsivity
  1. \<a\> \<b\>
  2. \<a\> \<b\>
  3. \< \>
  4. \<a\> \<b\>
  5. \< \>
  6. \<a\> \<b\>
  7. \< \>
  8. \<a\> \<b\>
  9. \<a\> \<b\> \<c\>
	1. \<a\> \<b\>
	2. \<a\> \<b\>
	3. \<a\> \<b\> \<c\> \<d\>
	4. \< \>
	5. \<a\> \<b\>
	6. \< \>
	7. \< \>
	8. \< \>
		1. \< \>
		2. \<a\> \<b\>
		3. \< \>
		4. \< \>
		5. \< \>
		6. \< \>
		7. \<a\> \<b\>
		8. \<a\> \<b\>
		9. \< \>
		10. \<a\> \<b\>
		11. \< \>
		12. \< \>
		13. \< \>
		14. \< \>
		15. \<a\> \<b\>

Criteria If ≥6 in *A only*, then criteria met Inattentive \< \> If ≥6 in *B only*, then criteria met Hyperactive–Impulsive \< \> If ≥6 in A *and* ≥6 in B, then criteria met Combined \< \>	**Criteria** If ≥4, then criteria met ODD \< \>	**Criteria** If ≥3, then criteria met CD \< \>

Duration
1. _____ (years old)
2. \< \> _____ (years old)
3. \< \> _____ (months)
 	
  * DUR met for ADHD \< \>
	Duration
	1. _____ (years old)
	2. \< \> _____ (years old)
	3. \< \> _____ (months)
	
	  * DUR met for ODD \< \>
		Duration
		1. _____ (years old)
		2. \< \> _____ (years old)
		3. \< \> _____ (months)
		
		  * DUR met for CD \< \>

Impairment 1. \< \> home 2. \< \> school 3. \< \> peers	**Impairment** 1. \< \> home 2. \< \> school 3. \< \> peers	**Impairment** 1. \< \> home 2. \< \> school 3. \< \> peers
		Type Childhood Onset \< \> Adolescent Onset \< \> Mild \< \> Moderate \< \> Severe \< \>

SUB AB	PHO	SOCIAL PHO

1. < >
    <a>_____
    <b>_____
    <c>_____
 	
    _____
2. < > _____
3. < > _____
4. < > _____
	1. _____
	   _____
	   _____
	2. <a> <b>
	3. <a> <b>
	4. <ai> <aii> <aiii> <aiv> <b>
	5. <a> <b>
		1. <a> <b>
		2. < >
		3. <a> <b>
		4. <ai> <aii> <aiii> <aiv> <b>
		5. < >

Duration	Criteria	Criteria

1. _____ (years old)
2. < > _____ (years old)
    _____ (months)
 	
  * DUR met for SUB AB < >
	If 1–4, then criteria met
	PHO < >
		If 1–4, then criteria met
		SOCIAL PHO < >

Duration	Duration
1. _____ (years old) 2. < > _____ (years old) 3. < > _____ (months) * DUR met for PHO < >	1. _____ (years old) 2. < > _____ (years old) 3. < > _____ (months) *DUR met for SOCIAL PHO < >

Impairment	Impairment	Impairment
1. <a> <b> 2. < > 3. <a> <b> 4. < >	1. < > home 2. < > school 3. < > peers	1. < > home 2. < > school 3. < > peers

Criteria	Type(s)
If any use (Q1–4) and any impairment (1–4), then criteria met SUB AB < >	Animal < > Natural Environment < > Blood–Injection–Injury < > Situational < > Other _____ < >

Type(s) _____
_____
_____
_____

SEP ANX	GEN ANX	OCD

1. <a> <b>
2. <a> <b>
3. < >
4. <a> <b>
5. <a> <b>
6. <a> <b>
7. <a> <b>
8. <a> <b>
	1. < > _____
	_____
	_____
	_____
	_____
	2. <a> <b>
	3. <a> <b> <c> <d> <e> <f>
		A. Compulsions
		   1. < > _____
		   2. <a> _____
		      <b>
		   3. < >
		
		B. Obsessions
		   1. <a> _____
		      <b> _____
		      <c> _____
		   2. <a> <b> <c>
		   3. < >
		
		C. Interference
		   1. <a> <b> <c>

Criteria
 	
   If ≥3, then criteria met
      SEP ANX < >
	Criteria
	
	   If 1–3, then criteria met
	      GEN ANX < >
		Criteria
		
		   If A1, A2, & C,
		   then criteria met
		   Compulsions < >
		
		   If B1, B2, & C,
		   then criteria met
		   Obsessions < >
		
		   If Compulsions +
		   and/or Obsessions +,
		   then criteria met
		   OCD < >

Duration 1. _____ (years old) 2. < > _____ (years old) 3. < > _____ (weeks) *DUR met for SEP ANX < >	**Duration** 1. _____ (years old) 2. < > _____ (years old) 3. < > _____ (months) *DUR met for GEN ANX < >	**Duration** 1. _____ (years old) 2. < > _____ (years old) _____ (months) *DUR met for OCD < >
Impairment 1. < > home 2. < > school 3. < > peers	**Impairment** 1. < > home 2. < > school 3. < > peers	**Impairment** 1. < > home 2. < > school 3. < > peers

STRESS (ASD/PTSD)	ANO	BUL
A. Exposure 　1. \<a> \<b> _____ 　2. \<a> \<b> \<c> \<d> \<e> 　3. \< > _____ B. Dissociation 　1. \<a> \<b> \<c> \<d> 　2. \< > 　3. \< > 　4. \< > 　5. \< > C. Reexperiencing 　1. \<a> \<b> \<c> 　2. \<a> \<b> 　3. \<a> \<b> 　4. \<a> \<b> 　5. \< > D. Avoidance 　1. \<a> \<b> 　2. \<a> \<b> \<c> 　3. \< > 　4. \<a> \<b> 　5. \<a> \<b> 　6. \<a> \<b> 　7. \<a> \<b> E. Hyperarousal 　1. \<a> \<b> 　2. \<a> \<b> 　3. \< > 　4. \< > 　5. \< >	1. \<a> \<b> 2. \<a> 　ht: _____ 　wt: _____ 　\<b> 　ht: _____ 　wt: _____ 3. \<a> \<b> \<c> 4. \<a> \<b> \<c> 5. \< >	1. \< > _____ _____ ⎯ 2. \<a> \<b> \<c> \<d> 3. \<a> \<b> \<c> \<d> 4. \<a> \<b>
Criteria If A1 & A2, ≥3 in B, ≥1 in C, ≥3 in D, and ≥2 in E, then criteria met ASD \< > If A1 & A2, ≥1 in C, ≥3 in D, and ≥2 in E, then criteria met PTSD \< >	**Criteria** If 1–4 (&5 for pubescent girls), then criteria met ANO \< >	**Criteria** If 1–4, then criteria met BUL \< >
Duration 1. _____ (years old) 2. \< > _____ (years old) 3. a. \< > _____ (weeks) 　b. \< > 　c. \< > _____ (days) 4. \< > _____ (months) 　　*DUR met for ASD \< > 　　*DUR met for PTSD \< >	**Duration** 1. _____ (years old) 2. \< > _____ (years old) 3. \< > _____ (months) 　*DUR met for ANO \< >	**Duration** 1. _____ (years old) 2. \< > _____ (years old) 3. a. \< > _____ (#/week) 　b. \< > _____ (months) 　*DUR met for BUL \< >
Impairment 1. \< > home 2. \< > school 3. \< > peers	**Impairment** 1. \< > home 2. \< > school 3. \< > peers	**Impairment** 1. \< > home 2. \< > school 3. \< > peers
Type (PTSD) Acute　　　\< > Regular Onset　\< > Chronic　　\< > Delayed Onset　\< >		

DEP/DYS (MDD/DD)	DEP/DYS (MDD/DD)	MAN/HYPOMAN

A. Dysphoric Mood
  1. \<a> \<b> \<c>
  2. \<a> \<bi> \<bii> \<biii>
    \<c> \<d>
 	
B. Loss of Interest
  1. \<a> \<b>
  2. \<a> \<b> \<c>
 	
C. Appetite Changes
  1. \<a> \<b> \<c>
  2. \<a> \<b>
 	
D. Sleep Changes
    Bedtime: _____
    Wakeup: _____
  1. \<a> \<b> \<c>
  2. \<a> \<b>
 	
E. Psychomotor Changes
  1. \<a> \<b> \<c> \<d>
  2. \<a> \<b>
 	
F. Low Energy
  1. \<a> \<b> \<c> \<d>
 	
G. Guilt
  1. \<a> \<b> \<c> \<d>
  2. \<a> \<b>
 	
H. Impaired Concentration
  1. \<a> \<b> \<c> \<d> \<e>
  2. \< >
 	
I. Hopelessness
  1. \<a> \<b> \<c>
 	
J. Morbid/Suicidal Thoughts
  1. \<a> \<b>
  2. \<a> \<b> \<c> \<d> \<e>
 	
_____
_____
_____
_____
_____
		A. Elevated Mood
		  1. \<a> _____
		    \<b> _____
		    \<c> _____
		  2. \< > _____
		
		B. Other Symptoms
		  1. \<a> _____
		    \<b>
		  2. \<a> \<b> \<c> _____
		  3. \<a> \<b> \<c> \<d>
		  4. \<a> \<b> \<c>
		  5. \< >
		  6. \<a> \<b> \<c> \<d> \<e>
		  7. \<a> \<b> \<c> \<d>
		
		C. Interference
		  1. \< >
		  2. \< >

	Criteria If A &/or B & ≥5 of A–H or J, then criteria met MDD \< > If A & ≥2 of C, D, F, G, H, or I, then criteria met DD \< >	**Criteria** If A1(a, b, & c) + ≥3 in B + ≥1 in C *or* A2 + ≥4 in B + ≥1 in C, then criteria met MAN \< > If A1(a, b, & c) + ≥3 in B + none in C *or* A2 + ≥4 in B + none in C, then criteria met HYPOMAN \< >

	Duration
	1. _____ (years old)
	2. \< > _____ (years old)
	3. MDD \< > _____ (weeks)
	   DD \< > _____ (months)
	
	  *DUR met for MDD \< >
	  *DUR met for DD \< >
		Duration
		1. _____ (years old)
		2. \< > _____ (years old)
		3. MAN \< > _____ (weeks)
		   HYPO \< > _____ (days)
		
		  *DUR met for MAN \< >
		  *DUR met for HYPOMAN \< >

	Impairment 1. \< > home 2. \< > school 3. \< > peers	**Impairment** 1. \< > home 2. \< > school 3. \< > peers

ENU	SCZ/PSY	STRESSORS

1. < >
2. <a> <b>
3. <a> <b>
 	
Criteria
If 1, ≥1 in 2, 3a, and 3b,
then criteria met
ENU < >
 	
Duration
1. _____ (years old)
2. < > _____ (years old)
3. <a> _____ (x/week)
   <b> _____ (months)
 	
  *DUR met for ENU < >
 	
Impairment
1. < > home
2. < > school
3. < > peers
	A. Psychotic Symptoms
	  1. <a> <b> <c> <d> <e>
	  2. <a> <b> <c> <d> <e> <f>
	  3. < >
	  4. < >
	  5. < >
	
	B. Interference
	  1. < >
	  2. < >
	  3. < >
		A. Child Abuse/Neglect
		1. <a> <b> <c>
		2. <a> <b> <c> <d>
		3. <a> <b> <c> <d>
		4. < >
		5. < >

		Duration 1. _____ 2. < > _____ 3. _____ 4. _____ 5. < >

Type
Nocturnal   < >
Diurnal   < >
Both   < >
	Criteria
	If ≥2 in A and ≥1 in B,
	then criteria met
	SCZ < >
	
	If ≥1 in A, then criteria met
	PSY < >
	
	Duration
	1. _____ (years old)
	2. < > _____ (years old)
	3. < > _____ (months)
	
	  *DUR met for SCZ < >
	  *DUR met for PSY < >
		B. Other Stressors
		  1. <a> <b> <c> <d> <e>
		  2. < >
		  3. <a> <b>
		  4. <a> <b> <c>
		  5. <a> <b>
		  6. <a> <b>
		  7. <a> _____
		      <b>
		  8. <a> <b> <c> <d>
		  9. < > _____
		      _____
		      _____
		10. < >
		11. < > _____
		      _____
		      _____

ENC		
1. < > 2. < > **Criteria** If both 1 & 2, then criteria met ENC < > **Duration** 1. _____ (years old) 2. < > _____ (years old) 3. <a> _____ (x/month) <b> _____ (months) *DUR met for ENC < > **Impairment** 1. < > home 2. < > school 3. < > peers	**Impairment** 1. < > home 2. < > school 3. < > peers	

ChIPS Scoring Form
Profile Sheet

Child's Number: _____ Date: _____

Child's Name: _____ Time Started: _____

Date of Birth: _____ Age: _____ Time Ended: _____

Race: _____ Sex: _____ Interviewer: _____

Setting (circle one): Inpatient, Outpatient, School, Other Research Setting: _____

	Disorder	Symptoms	Diagnosis	Duration	Clinician's Diagnosis
ADHD	**Attention-Deficit/Hyperactivity Disorder**	<>	<>	<>	Axis I
	Type: Inattentive, Hyperactive–Impulsive, Combined				
ODD	**Oppositional Defiant Disorder**	<>	<>	<>	
CD	**Conduct Disorder**	<>	<>	<>	
	Onset: Childhood, Adolescent				
	Severity: Mild, Moderate, Severe				
SUBAB	**Substance Abuse**	<>	<>	<>	
	Substance(s): _____				
PHO	**Specific Phobia**	<>	<>	<>	Axis II
	Type: _____				
SOCPHO	**Social Phobia**	<>	<>	<>	
SEPANX	**Separation Anxiety Disorder**	<>	<>	<>	Axis III
GENANX	**General Anxiety Disorder**	<>	<>	<>	
OCD	**Obsessive-Compulsive Disorder**	<>	<>	<>	
PTSD	**Posttraumatic Stress Disorder**	<>	<>	<>	Axis IV
	Type: Acute, Chronic				
	Onset: Regular, Delayed				
ASD	**Acute Stress Disorder**	<>	<>	<>	
ANO	**Anorexia**	<>	<>	<>	Axis V
BUL	**Bulimia**	<>	<>	<>	current:
DEP	**Major Depressive Disorder**	<>	<>	<>	past year:
DYS	**Dysthymic Disorder**	<>	<>	<>	
MAN	**Mania**	<>	<>	<>	
HYPOMAN	**Hypomania**	<>	<>	<>	
ENU	**Enuresis**	<>	<>	<>	
	Type: Nocturnal, Diurnal, Both				
ENC	**Encopresis**	<>	<>	<>	
SCZ	**Schizophrenia**	<>	<>	<>	
PSY	**Psychosis**	<>	<>	<>	

Psychosocial Stressors:

Other Stressors:

Behavioral Observations

Appearance: Affect:

Effort: Level of Activity:

Unusual Behaviors:

Presenting Problem

Home

1.

2.

School

1.

2.

3.

4.

5.

Peers/Work

1.

2.

3.

4.

5.

Medication

Type:

Dosage:

Child's Name: _____

Date: _____

ADHD	ODD	CD

A. Inattention
  1. <a> <b>
  2. < >
  3. <a> <b>
  4. <a> <b> <c>
  5. < >
  6. < >
  7. < >
  8. <a> <b>
  9. <a> <b>
 	
B. Hyperactivity–Impulsivity
  1. <a> <b>
  2. <a> <b>
  3. < >
  4. <a> <b>
  5. < >
  6. <a> <b>
  7. < >
  8. <a> <b>
  9. <a> <b> <c>
	1. <a> <b>
	2. <a> <b>
	3. <a> <b> <c> <d>
	4. < >
	5. <a> <b>
	6. < >
	7. < >
	8. < >
		1. < >
		2. <a> <b>
		3. < >
		4. < >
		5. < >
		6. < >
		7. <a> <b>
		8. <a> <b>
		9. < >
		10. <a> <b>
		11. < >
		12. < >
		13. < >
		14. < >
		15. <a> <b>

Criteria If ≥6 in *A only*, then criteria met Inattentive < > If ≥6 in *B only*, then criteria met Hyperactive–Impulsive < > If ≥6 in A *and* ≥6 in B, then criteria met Combined < >	**Criteria** If ≥4, then criteria met ODD < >	**Criteria** If ≥3, then criteria met CD < >

Duration
1. _____ (years old)
2. < > _____ (years old)
3. < > _____ (months)
 	
  * DUR met for ADHD < >
	Duration
	1. _____ (years old)
	2. < > _____ (years old)
	3. < > _____ (months)
	
	  * DUR met for ODD < >
		Duration
		1. _____ (years old)
		2. < > _____ (years old)
		3. < > _____ (months)
		
		  * DUR met for CD < >

Impairment 1. < > home 2. < > school 3. < > peers	**Impairment** 1. < > home 2. < > school 3. < > peers	**Impairment** 1. < > home 2. < > school 3. < > peers
		Type Childhood Onset < > Adolescent Onset < > Mild < > Moderate < > Severe < >

SUB AB	PHO	SOCIAL PHO
1. < > <a>_____ <b>_____ <c>_____ _____ 2. < > _____ 3. < > _____ 4. < > _____	1. _____ _____ _____ 2. <a> <b> 3. <a> <b> 4. <ai> <aii> <aiii> <aiv> <b> 5. <a> <b>	1. <a> <b> 2. < > 3. <a> <b> 4. <ai> <aii> <aiii> <aiv> <b> 5. < >
Duration 1. _____ (years old) 2. < > _____ (years old) _____ (months) * DUR met for SUB AB < >	**Criteria** If 1–4, then criteria met PHO < >	**Criteria** If 1–4, then criteria met SOCIAL PHO < >
	Duration 1. _____ (years old) 2. < > _____ (years old) 3. < > _____ (months) * DUR met for PHO < >	**Duration** 1. _____ (years old) 2. < > _____ (years old) 3. < > _____ (months) *DUR met for SOCIAL PHO < >
Impairment 1. <a> <b> 2. < > 3. <a> <b> 4. < >	**Impairment** 1. < > home 2. < > school 3. < > peers	**Impairment** 1. < > home 2. < > school 3. < > peers
Criteria If any use (Q1–4) and any impairment (1–4), then criteria met SUB AB < > **Type(s)** _____ _____ _____ _____	**Type(s)** Animal < > Natural Environment < > Blood–Injection–Injury < > Situational < > Other _____ < >	

SEP ANX	GEN ANX	OCD

1. \<a\> \<b\>
2. \<a\> \<b\>
3. \< \>
4. \<a\> \<b\>
5. \<a\> \<b\>
6. \<a\> \<b\>
7. \<a\> \<b\>
8. \<a\> \<b\>
	1. \< \> _____
	  _____
	  _____
	  _____
	  _____
	2. \<a\> \<b\>
	3. \<a\> \<b\> \<c\> \<d\> \<e\> \<f\>
		A. Compulsions
		  1. \< \> _____
		  2. \<a\> _____
		   \<b\>
		  3. \< \>
		
		B. Obsessions
		  1. \<a\> _____
		   \<b\> _____
		   \<c\> _____
		  2. \<a\> \<b\> \<c\>
		  3. \< \>
		
		C. Interference
		  1. \<a\> \<b\> \<c\>

Criteria
  If ≥3, then criteria met
  SEP ANX \< \>
	Criteria
	  If 1–3, then criteria met
	  GEN ANX \< \>
		Criteria
		  If A1, A2, & C,
		  then criteria met
		  Compulsions \< \>
		
		  If B1, B2, & C,
		  then criteria met
		  Obsessions \< \>
		
		  If Compulsions +
		  and/or Obsessions +,
		  then criteria met
		  OCD \< \>

Duration
1. _____ (years old)
2. \< \> _____ (years old)
3. \< \> _____ (weeks)
 	
  *DUR met for SEP ANX \< \>
	Duration
	1. _____ (years old)
	2. \< \> _____ (years old)
	3. \< \> _____ (months)
	
	  *DUR met for GEN ANX \< \>
		Duration
		1. _____ (years old)
		2. \< \> _____ (years old)
		  _____ (months)
		
		  *DUR met for OCD \< \>

Impairment 1. \< \> home 2. \< \> school 3. \< \> peers	**Impairment** 1. \< \> home 2. \< \> school 3. \< \> peers	**Impairment** 1. \< \> home 2. \< \> school 3. \< \> peers

STRESS (ASD/PTSD)	ANO	BUL

A. Exposure
  1. <a> <b> _____
  2. <a> <b> <c> <d> <e>
  3. < > _____
B. Dissociation
  1. <a> <b> <c> <d>
  2. < >
  3. < >
  4. < >
  5. < >
C. Reexperiencing
  1. <a> <b> <c>
  2. <a> <b>
  3. <a> <b>
  4. <a> <b>
  5. < >
D. Avoidance
  1. <a> <b>
  2. <a> <b> <c>
  3. < >
  4. <a> <b>
  5. <a> <b>
  6. <a> <b>
  7. <a> <b>
E. Hyperarousal
  1. <a> <b>
  2. <a> <b>
  3. < >
  4. < >
  5. < >
	1. <a> <b>
	2. <a>
	  ht: _____
	  wt: _____
	  <b>
	  ht: _____
	  wt: _____
	3. <a> <b> <c>
	4. <a> <b> <c>
	5. < >
		1. < > _____
		_____
		2. <a> <b> <c> <d>
		3. <a> <b> <c> <d>
		4. <a> <b>

Criteria If A1 & A2, ≥3 in B, ≥1 in C, ≥3 in D, and ≥2 in E, then criteria met ASD < > If A1 & A2, ≥1 in C, ≥3 in D, and ≥2 in E, then criteria met PTSD < >	**Criteria** If 1–4 (&5 for pubescent girls), then criteria met ANO < >	**Criteria** If 1–4, then criteria met BUL < >

Duration
1. _____ (years old)
2. < > _____ (years old)
3. a. < > _____ (weeks)
   b. < >
   c. < > _____ (days)
4. < > _____ (months)
    *DUR met for ASD < >
    *DUR met for PTSD < >
	Duration
	1. _____ (years old)
	2. < > _____ (years old)
	3. < > _____ (months)
	
	   *DUR met for ANO < >
		Duration
		1. _____ (years old)
		2. < > _____ (years old)
		3. a. < > _____ (#/week)
		   b. < > _____ (months)
		
		   *DUR met for BUL < >

Impairment 1. < > home 2. < > school 3. < > peers	**Impairment** 1. < > home 2. < > school 3. < > peers	**Impairment** 1. < > home 2. < > school 3. < > peers
Type (PTSD) Acute < > Regular Onset < > Chronic < > Delayed Onset < >		

DEP/DYS (MDD/DD)	DEP/DYS (MDD/DD)	MAN/HYPOMAN

A. Dysphoric Mood
  1. \<a> \<b> \<c>
  2. \<a> \<bi> \<bii> \<biii>
    \<c> \<d>
 	
B. Loss of Interest
  1. \<a> \<b>
  2. \<a> \<b> \<c>
 	
C. Appetite Changes
  1. \<a> \<b> \<c>
  2. \<a> \<b>
 	
D. Sleep Changes
    Bedtime: _____
    Wakeup: _____
  1. \<a> \<b> \<c>
  2. \<a> \<b>
 	
E. Psychomotor Changes
  1. \<a> \<b> \<c> \<d>
  2. \<a> \<b>
 	
F. Low Energy
  1. \<a> \<b> \<c> \<d>
 	
G. Guilt
  1. \<a> \<b> \<c> \<d>
  2. \<a> \<b>
 	
H. Impaired Concentration
  1. \<a> \<b> \<c> \<d> \<e>
  2. \< >
 	
I. Hopelessness
  1. \<a> \<b> \<c>
 	
J. Morbid/Suicidal Thoughts
  1. \<a> \<b>
  2. \<a> \<b> \<c> \<d> \<e>
 	
_____
_____
_____
_____
_____
		A. Elevated Mood
		  1. \<a> _____
		    \<b> _____
		    \<c> _____
		  2. \< > _____
		
		B. Other Symptoms
		  1. \<a> _____
		    \<b>
		  2. \<a> \<b> \<c> _____
		  3. \<a> \<b> \<c> \<d>
		  4. \<a> \<b> \<c>
		  5. \< >
		  6. \<a> \<b> \<c> \<d> \<e>
		  7. \<a> \<b> \<c> \<d>
		
		C. Interference
		  1. \< >
		  2. \< >

	Criteria If A &/or B & ≥5 of A–H or J, then criteria met MDD \< > If A & ≥2 of C, D, F, G, H, or I, then criteria met DD \< >	**Criteria** If A1(a, b, & c) + ≥3 in B + ≥1 in C *or* A2 + ≥4 in B + ≥1 in C, then criteria met MAN \< > If A1(a, b, & c) + ≥3 in B + none in C *or* A2 + ≥4 in B + none in C, then criteria met HYPOMAN \< >

	Duration
	1. _____ (years old)
	2. \< > _____ (years old)
	3. MDD \< > _____ (weeks)
	   DD \< > _____ (months)
	
	*DUR met for MDD \< >
	*DUR met for DD \< >
		Duration
		1. _____ (years old)
		2. \< > _____ (years old)
		3. MAN \< > _____ (weeks)
		   HYPO \< > _____ (days)
		
		*DUR met for MAN \< >
		*DUR met for HYPOMAN \< >

	Impairment 1. \< > home 2. \< > school 3. \< > peers	**Impairment** 1. \< > home 2. \< > school 3. \< > peers

ENU	SCZ/PSY	STRESSORS

1. < >
 2. \<a> \<b>
 3. \<a> \<b>
	A. Psychotic Symptoms
	   1. \<a> \<b> \<c> \<d> \<e>
	   2. \<a> \<b> \<c> \<d> \<e> \<f>
	   3. < >
	   4. < >
	   5. < >
		A. Child Abuse/Neglect
		   1. \<a> \<b> \<c>
		   2. \<a> \<b> \<c> \<d>
		   3. \<a> \<b> \<c> \<d>
		   4. < >
		   5. < >

Criteria
   If 1, ≥1 in 2, 3a, and 3b,
     then criteria met
       ENU < >
	B. Interference
	   1. < >
	   2. < >
	   3. < >
		Duration
		   1. _____
		   2. < > _____
		   3. _____
		   4. _____
		   5. < >

Duration
 1. _____ (years old)
 2. < > _____ (years old)
 3. \<a> _____ (x/week)
    \<b> _____ (months)
 	
   *DUR met for ENU < >
	Criteria
	   If ≥2 in A and ≥1 in B,
	     then criteria met
	       SCZ < >
	
	   If ≥1 in A, then criteria met
	       PSY < >
		B. Other Stressors
		   1. \<a> \<b> \<c> \<d> \<e>
		   2. < >
		   3. \<a> \<b>
		   4. \<a> \<b> \<c>
		   5. \<a> \<b>
		   6. \<a> \<b>
		   7. \<a> _____
		      \<b>
		   8. \<a> \<b> \<c> \<d>
		   9. < > _____

Impairment
 1. < > home
 2. < > school
 3. < > peers
	Duration
	 1. _____ (years old)
	 2. < > _____ (years old)
	 3. < > _____ (months)
	
	   *DUR met for SCZ < >
	   *DUR met for PSY < >
		_____
		 _____
		   10. < >
		   11. < > _____

Type Nocturnal < > Diurnal < > Both < >		_____ _____
ENC	**Impairment** 1. < > home 2. < > school 3. < > peers	
1. < > 2. < >		
Criteria If both 1 & 2, then criteria met ENC < >		

Duration
 1. _____ (years old)
 2. < > _____ (years old)
 3. \<a> _____ (x/month)
    \<b> _____ (months)
 	
   *DUR met for ENC < >		

Impairment 1. < > home 2. < > school 3. < > peers		

ChIPS Scoring Form
Profile Sheet

Child's Number: _____   Date: _____

Child's Name: _____   Time Started: _____

Date of Birth: _____ Age: _____   Time Ended: _____

Race: _____ Sex: _____   Interviewer: _____

Setting (circle one):   Inpatient,   Outpatient,   School,   Other Research Setting: _____

	Disorder	Symptoms	Diagnosis	Duration	Clinician's Diagnosis
ADHD	**Attention-Deficit/Hyperactivity Disorder**	<>	<>	<>	Axis I
	Type: Inattentive, Hyperactive–Impulsive, Combined				
ODD	**Oppositional Defiant Disorder**	<>	<>	<>	
CD	**Conduct Disorder**	<>	<>	<>	
	Onset: Childhood, Adolescent				
	Severity: Mild, Moderate, Severe				
SUBAB	**Substance Abuse**	<>	<>	<>	
	Substance(s): _____				
PHO	**Specific Phobia**	<>	<>	<>	Axis II
	Type: _____				
SOCPHO	**Social Phobia**	<>	<>	<>	
SEPANX	**Separation Anxiety Disorder**	<>	<>	<>	Axis III
GENANX	**General Anxiety Disorder**	<>	<>	<>	
OCD	**Obsessive-Compulsive Disorder**	<>	<>	<>	
PTSD	**Posttraumatic Stress Disorder**	<>	<>	<>	Axis IV
	Type: Acute, Chronic				
	Onset: Regular, Delayed				
ASD	**Acute Stress Disorder**	<>	<>	<>	
ANO	**Anorexia**	<>	<>	<>	Axis V
BUL	**Bulimia**	<>	<>	<>	current:
DEP	**Major Depressive Disorder**	<>	<>	<>	past year:
DYS	**Dysthymic Disorder**	<>	<>	<>	
MAN	**Mania**	<>	<>	<>	
HYPOMAN	**Hypomania**	<>	<>	<>	
ENU	**Enuresis**	<>	<>	<>	
	Type: Nocturnal, Diurnal, Both				
ENC	**Encopresis**	<>	<>	<>	
SCZ	**Schizophrenia**	<>	<>	<>	
PSY	**Psychosis**	<>	<>	<>	

Psychosocial Stressors:

Other Stressors:

Behavioral Observations

Appearance: Affect:

Effort: Level of Activity:

Unusual Behaviors:

Presenting Problem

Home

1.

2.

School

1.

2.

3.

4.

5.

Peers/Work

1.

2.

3.

4.

5.

Medication

Type:

Dosage:

Child's Name: _____

Date: _____

ADHD	ODD	CD
A. Inattention 1. \<a\> \<b\> 2. \< \> 3. \<a\> \<b\> 4. \<a\> \<b\> \<c\> 5. \< \> 6. \< \> 7. \< \> 8. \<a\> \<b\> 9. \<a\> \<b\> B. Hyperactivity–Impulsivity 1. \<a\> \<b\> 2. \<a\> \<b\> 3. \< \> 4. \<a\> \<b\> 5. \< \> 6. \<a\> \<b\> 7. \< \> 8. \<a\> \<b\> 9. \<a\> \<b\> \<c\>	1. \<a\> \<b\> 2. \<a\> \<b\> 3. \<a\> \<b\> \<c\> \<d\> 4. \< \> 5. \<a\> \<b\> 6. \< \> 7. \< \> 8. \< \>	1. \< \> 2. \<a\> \<b\> 3. \< \> 4. \< \> 5. \< \> 6. \< \> 7. \<a\> \<b\> 8. \<a\> \<b\> 9. \< \> 10. \<a\> \<b\> 11. \< \> 12. \< \> 13. \< \> 14. \< \> 15. \<a\> \<b\>
Criteria If ≥6 in *A only*, then criteria met Inattentive \< \> If ≥6 in *B only*, then criteria met Hyperactive–Impulsive \< \> If ≥6 in A *and* ≥6 in B, then criteria met Combined \< \>	**Criteria** If ≥4, then criteria met ODD \< \>	**Criteria** If ≥3, then criteria met CD \< \>

Duration
1. _____ (years old)
2. \< \> _____ (years old)
3. \< \> _____ (months)
 	
    * DUR met for ADHD \< \>
	Duration
	1. _____ (years old)
	2. \< \> _____ (years old)
	3. \< \> _____ (months)
	
	    * DUR met for ODD \< \>
		Duration
		1. _____ (years old)
		2. \< \> _____ (years old)
		3. \< \> _____ (months)
		
		    * DUR met for CD \< \>

Impairment 1. \< \> home 2. \< \> school 3. \< \> peers	**Impairment** 1. \< \> home 2. \< \> school 3. \< \> peers	**Impairment** 1. \< \> home 2. \< \> school 3. \< \> peers
		Type Childhood Onset \< \> Adolescent Onset \< \> Mild \< \> Moderate \< \> Severe \< \>

SUB AB	PHO	SOCIAL PHO

1. < >
    <a>_____
    <b>_____
    <c>_____
 	
    _____
2. < > _____
3. < > _____
4. < > _____
	1. _____
	    _____
	    _____
	2. <a> <b>
	3. <a> <b>
	4. <ai> <aii> <aiii> <aiv> <b>
	5. <a> <b>
		1. <a> <b>
		2. < >
		3. <a> <b>
		4. <ai> <aii> <aiii> <aiv> <b>
		5. < >

Duration
1. _____ (years old)
2. < > _____ (years old)
    _____ (months)
 	
  * DUR met for SUB AB < >
	Criteria
	    If 1–4, then criteria met
	        PHO < >
		Criteria
		    If 1–4, then criteria met
		      SOCIAL PHO < >

	Duration
	1. _____ (years old)
	2. < > _____ (years old)
	3. < > _____ (months)
	
	    * DUR met for PHO < >
		Duration
		1. _____ (years old)
		2. < > _____ (years old)
		3. < > _____ (months)
		
		    *DUR met for SOCIAL PHO < >

Impairment 1. <a> <b> 2. < > 3. <a> <b> 4. < >	**Impairment** 1. < > home 2. < > school 3. < > peers	**Impairment** 1. < > home 2. < > school 3. < > peers

Criteria
    If any use (Q1–4) and any
  impairment (1–4), then criteria
      met SUB AB < >
 	
Type(s) _____
_____
_____
_____
	Type(s)
	Animal < >
	Natural Environment < >
	Blood–Injection–Injury < >
	Situational < >
	Other _____ < >	

SEP ANX	GEN ANX	OCD

1. \<a\> \<b\>
2. \<a\> \<b\>
3. \< \>
4. \<a\> \<b\>
5. \<a\> \<b\>
6. \<a\> \<b\>
7. \<a\> \<b\>
8. \<a\> \<b\>
	1. \< \> _____
	_____
	_____
	_____
	_____
	2. \<a\> \<b\>
	3. \<a\> \<b\> \<c\> \<d\> \<e\> \<f\>
		A. Compulsions
		  1. \< \> _____
		  2. \<a\> _____
		     \<b\>
		  3. \< \>
		
		B. Obsessions
		  1. \<a\> _____
		     \<b\> _____
		     \<c\> _____
		  2. \<a\> \<b\> \<c\>
		  3. \< \>
		
		C. Interference
		  1. \<a\> \<b\> \<c\>

Criteria
  If ≥3, then criteria met
    SEP ANX \< \>
	Criteria
	  If 1–3, then criteria met
	    GEN ANX \< \>
		Criteria
		  If A1, A2, & C,
		  then criteria met
		  Compulsions \< \>
		
		  If B1, B2, & C,
		  then criteria met
		  Obsessions \< \>
		
		  If Compulsions +
		  and/or Obsessions +,
		  then criteria met
		  OCD \< \>

Duration
1. _____ (years old)
2. \< \> _____ (years old)
3. \< \> _____ (weeks)
 	
  *DUR met for SEP ANX \< \>
	Duration
	1. _____ (years old)
	2. \< \> _____ (years old)
	3. \< \> _____ (months)
	
	  *DUR met for GEN ANX \< \>
		Duration
		1. _____ (years old)
		2. \< \> _____ (years old)
		    _____ (months)
		
		  *DUR met for OCD \< \>

Impairment 1. \< \> home 2. \< \> school 3. \< \> peers	**Impairment** 1. \< \> home 2. \< \> school 3. \< \> peers	**Impairment** 1. \< \> home 2. \< \> school 3. \< \> peers

STRESS (ASD/PTSD)	ANO	BUL

A. Exposure
  1. \<a> \<b> _____
  2. \<a> \<b> \<c> \<d> \<e>
  3. \< > _____
B. Dissociation
  1. \<a> \<b> \<c> \<d>
  2. \< >
  3. \< >
  4. \< >
  5. \< >
C. Reexperiencing
  1. \<a> \<b> \<c>
  2. \<a> \<b>
  3. \<a> \<b>
  4. \<a> \<b>
  5. \< >
D. Avoidance
  1. \<a> \<b>
  2. \<a> \<b> \<c>
  3. \< >
  4. \<a> \<b>
  5. \<a> \<b>
  6. \<a> \<b>
  7. \<a> \<b>
E. Hyperarousal
  1. \<a> \<b>
  2. \<a> \<b>
  3. \< >
  4. \< >
  5. \< >
	1. \<a> \<b>
	2. \<a>
	  ht: _____
	  wt: _____
	  \<b>
	  ht: _____
	  wt: _____
	3. \<a> \<b> \<c>
	4. \<a> \<b> \<c>
	5. \< >
		1. \< > _____
		
		_____
		2. \<a> \<b> \<c> \<d>
		3. \<a> \<b> \<c> \<d>
		4. \<a> \<b>

Criteria If A1 & A2, ≥3 in B, ≥1 in C, ≥3 in D, and ≥2 in E, then criteria met ASD \< > If A1 & A2, ≥1 in C, ≥3 in D, and ≥2 in E, then criteria met PTSD \< >	**Criteria** If 1–4 (&5 for pubescent girls), then criteria met ANO \< >	**Criteria** If 1–4, then criteria met BUL \< >

Duration
1. _____ (years old)
2. \< > _____ (years old)
3. a. \< > _____ (weeks)
   b. \< >
   c. \< > _____ (days)
4. \< > _____ (months)
    *DUR met for ASD \< >
    *DUR met for PTSD \< >
	Duration
	1. _____ (years old)
	2. \< > _____ (years old)
	3. \< > _____ (months)
	
	   *DUR met for ANO \< >
		Duration
		1. _____ (years old)
		2. \< > _____ (years old)
		3. a. \< > _____ (#/week)
		   b. \< > _____ (months)
		
		   *DUR met for BUL \< >

Impairment 1. \< > home 2. \< > school 3. \< > peers	**Impairment** 1. \< > home 2. \< > school 3. \< > peers	**Impairment** 1. \< > home 2. \< > school 3. \< > peers
Type (PTSD) Acute \< > Regular Onset \< > Chronic \< > Delayed Onset \< >		

DEP/DYS (MDD/DD)	DEP/DYS (MDD/DD)	MAN/HYPOMAN

A. Dysphoric Mood
  1. \<a> \<b> \<c>
  2. \<a> \<bi> \<bii> \<biii>
    \<c> \<d>
 	
B. Loss of Interest
  1. \<a> \<b>
  2. \<a> \<b> \<c>
 	
C. Appetite Changes
  1. \<a> \<b> \<c>
  2. \<a> \<b>
 	
D. Sleep Changes
    Bedtime: _____
    Wakeup: _____
  1. \<a> \<b> \<c>
  2. \<a> \<b>
 	
E. Psychomotor Changes
  1. \<a> \<b> \<c> \<d>
  2. \<a> \<b>
 	
F. Low Energy
  1. \<a> \<b> \<c> \<d>
 	
G. Guilt
  1. \<a> \<b> \<c> \<d>
  2. \<a> \<b>
 	
H. Impaired Concentration
  1. \<a> \<b> \<c> \<d> \<e>
  2. \< >
 	
I. Hopelessness
  1. \<a> \<b> \<c>
 	
J. Morbid/Suicidal Thoughts
  1. \<a> \<b>
  2. \<a> \<b> \<c> \<d> \<e>
 	
_____
_____
_____
_____
_____
		A. Elevated Mood
		  1. \<a> _____
		    \<b> _____
		    \<c> _____
		  2. \< > _____
		
		B. Other Symptoms
		  1. \<a> _____
		    \<b>
		  2. \<a> \<b> \<c> _____
		  3. \<a> \<b> \<c> \<d>
		  4. \<a> \<b> \<c>
		  5. \< >
		  6. \<a> \<b> \<c> \<d> \<e>
		  7. \<a> \<b> \<c> \<d>
		
		C. Interference
		  1. \< >
		  2. \< >

	Criteria
	  If A &/or B & ≥5 of A–H or J,
	    then criteria met
	      MDD \< >
	
	  If A & ≥2 of C, D, F, G, H, or I,
	    then criteria met
	      DD \< >
		Criteria
		  If A1(a, b, & c) + ≥3 in B + ≥1 in C
		      or
		  A2 + ≥4 in B + ≥1 in C,
		    then criteria met
		      MAN \< >
		
		  If A1(a, b, & c) + ≥3 in B +
		    none in C
		      or
		  A2 + ≥4 in B + none in C,
		    then criteria met
		      HYPOMAN \< >

	Duration
	  1. _____ (years old)
	  2. \< > _____ (years old)
	  3. MDD \< > _____ (weeks)
	    DD \< > _____ (months)
	
	    *DUR met for MDD \< >
	    *DUR met for DD \< >
		Duration
		  1. _____ (years old)
		  2. \< > _____ (years old)
		  3. MAN \< > _____ (weeks)
		    HYPO \< > _____ (days)
		
		    *DUR met for MAN \< >
		    *DUR met for HYPOMAN \< >

	Impairment
	  1. \< > home
	  2. \< > school
	  3. \< > peers
		Impairment
		  1. \< > home
		  2. \< > school
		  3. \< > peers

ENU	SCZ/PSY	STRESSORS

1. < >
 2. <a> <b>
 3. <a> <b>
	A. Psychotic Symptoms
	    1. <a> <b> <c> <d> <e>
	    2. <a> <b> <c> <d> <e> <f>
	    3. < >
	    4. < >
	    5. < >
		A. Child Abuse/Neglect
		    1. <a> <b> <c>
		    2. <a> <b> <c> <d>
		    3. <a> <b> <c> <d>
		    4. < >
		    5. < >

Criteria
    If 1, ≥1 in 2, 3a, and 3b,
      then criteria met
        ENU < >
	B. Interference
	    1. < >
	    2. < >
	    3. < >
		Duration
		    1. _____
		    2. < > _____
		    3. _____
		    4. _____
		    5. < >

Duration
    1. _____ (years old)
    2. < > _____ (years old)
    3. <a> _____ (x/week)
      <b> _____ (months)
 	
    *DUR met for ENU < >
	Criteria
	    If ≥2 in A and ≥1 in B,
	      then criteria met
	        SCZ < >
	
	    If ≥1 in A, then criteria met
	        PSY < >
		B. Other Stressors
		    1. <a> <b> <c> <d> <e>
		    2. < >
		    3. <a> <b>
		    4. <a> <b> <c>
		    5. <a> <b>
		    6. <a> <b>
		    7. <a> _____
		        <b>
		    8. <a> <b> <c> <d>
		    9. < > _____

Impairment
    1. < > home
    2. < > school
    3. < > peers
	Duration
	    1. _____ (years old)
	    2. < > _____ (years old)
	    3. < > _____ (months)
	
	    *DUR met for SCZ < >
	    *DUR met for PSY < >
		_____
		    10. < > _____
		    11. < > _____
		 _____
		 _____

Type Nocturnal < > Diurnal < > Both < >		

ENC	**Impairment**
	    1. < > home
	    2. < > school
	    3. < > peers	

1. < > 2. < >		
Criteria If both 1 & 2, then criteria met ENC < >		

Duration
    1. _____ (years old)
    2. < > _____ (years old)
    3. <a> _____ (x/month)
      <b> _____ (months)
 	
    *DUR met for ENC < >		

Impairment
    1. < > home
    2. < > school
    3. < > peers		

ChIPS Scoring Form
Profile Sheet

Child's Number: _____   Date: _____

Child's Name: _____   Time Started: _____

Date of Birth: _____ Age: _____   Time Ended: _____

Race: _____ Sex: _____   Interviewer: _____

Setting (circle one):   Inpatient,   Outpatient,   School,   Other Research Setting: _____

	Disorder	Symptoms	Diagnosis	Duration	Clinician's Diagnosis
ADHD	**Attention-Deficit/Hyperactivity Disorder** *Type:* Inattentive, Hyperactive–Impulsive, Combined	<>	<>	<>	**Axis I**
ODD	**Oppositional Defiant Disorder**	<>	<>	<>	
CD	**Conduct Disorder** *Onset:* Childhood, Adolescent *Severity:* Mild, Moderate, Severe	<>	<>	<>	
SUBAB	**Substance Abuse** *Substance(s):* _____	<>	<>	<>	
PHO	**Specific Phobia** *Type:* _____	<>	<>	<>	**Axis II**
SOCPHO	**Social Phobia**	<>	<>	<>	
SEPANX	**Separation Anxiety Disorder**	<>	<>	<>	**Axis III**
GENANX	**General Anxiety Disorder**	<>	<>	<>	
OCD	**Obsessive-Compulsive Disorder**	<>	<>	<>	
PTSD	**Posttraumatic Stress Disorder** *Type:* Acute, Chronic *Onset:* Regular, Delayed	<>	<>	<>	**Axis IV**
ASD	**Acute Stress Disorder**	<>	<>	<>	
ANO	**Anorexia**	<>	<>	<>	**Axis V**
BUL	**Bulimia**	<>	<>	<>	current:
DEP	**Major Depressive Disorder**	<>	<>	<>	past year:
DYS	**Dysthymic Disorder**	<>	<>	<>	
MAN	**Mania**	<>	<>	<>	
HYPOMAN	**Hypomania**	<>	<>	<>	
ENU	**Enuresis** *Type:* Nocturnal, Diurnal, Both	<>	<>	<>	
ENC	**Encopresis**	<>	<>	<>	
SCZ	**Schizophrenia**	<>	<>	<>	
PSY	**Psychosis**	<>	<>	<>	

Psychosocial Stressors:

Other Stressors:

Behavioral Observations

Appearance: Affect:

Effort: Level of Activity:

Unusual Behaviors:

Presenting Problem

Home

1.

2.

School

1.

2.

3.

4.

5.

Peers/Work

1.

2.

3.

4.

5.

Medication

Type:

Dosage:

Child's Name: _____

Date: _____

ADHD	ODD	CD

A. Inattention
  1. <a> <b>
  2. < >
  3. <a> <b>
  4. <a> <b> <c>
  5. < >
  6. < >
  7. < >
  8. <a> <b>
  9. <a> <b>
 	
B. Hyperactivity–Impulsivity
  1. <a> <b>
  2. <a> <b>
  3. < >
  4. <a> <b>
  5. < >
  6. <a> <b>
  7. < >
  8. <a> <b>
  9. <a> <b> <c>
	1. <a> <b>
	2. <a> <b>
	3. <a> <b> <c> <d>
	4. < >
	5. <a> <b>
	6. < >
	7. < >
	8. < >
		1. < >
		2. <a> <b>
		3. < >
		4. < >
		5. < >
		6. < >
		7. <a> <b>
		8. <a> <b>
		9. < >
		10. <a> <b>
		11. < >
		12. < >
		13. < >
		14. < >
		15. <a> <b>

Criteria If ≥6 in *A only*, then criteria met Inattentive < > If ≥6 in *B only*, then criteria met Hyperactive–Impulsive < > If ≥6 in A *and* ≥6 in B, then criteria met Combined < >	**Criteria** If ≥4, then criteria met ODD < >	**Criteria** If ≥3, then criteria met CD < >

Duration
1. _____ (years old)
2. < > _____ (years old)
3. < > _____ (months)
 	
  * DUR met for ADHD < >
	Duration
	1. _____ (years old)
	2. < > _____ (years old)
	3. < > _____ (months)
	
	  * DUR met for ODD < >
		Duration
		1. _____ (years old)
		2. < > _____ (years old)
		3. < > _____ (months)
		
		  * DUR met for CD < >

Impairment 1. < > home 2. < > school 3. < > peers	**Impairment** 1. < > home 2. < > school 3. < > peers	**Impairment** 1. < > home 2. < > school 3. < > peers
		Type Childhood Onset < > Adolescent Onset < > Mild < > Moderate < > Severe < >

SUB AB	PHO	SOCIAL PHO

1. < >
     <a>_____
     <b>_____
     <c>_____
 	
     _____
 2. < > _____
 3. < > _____
 4. < > _____
	1. _____
	    _____
	    _____
	 2. <a> <b>
	 3. <a> <b>
	 4. <ai> <aii> <aiii> <aiv> <b>
	 5. <a> <b>
		1. <a> <b>
		 2. < >
		 3. <a> <b>
		 4. <ai> <aii> <aiii> <aiv> <b>
		 5. < >

Duration (SUB AB)

1. _____ (years old)
2. < > _____ (years old)
   _____ (months)

   * DUR met for SUB AB < >

Criteria (PHO)

   If 1–4, then criteria met
      PHO < >

Criteria (SOCIAL PHO)

   If 1–4, then criteria met
    SOCIAL PHO < >

Duration (PHO)

1. _____ (years old)
2. < > _____ (years old)
3. < > _____ (months)

   * DUR met for PHO < >

Duration (SOCIAL PHO)

1. _____ (years old)
2. < > _____ (years old)
3. < > _____ (months)

   *DUR met for SOCIAL PHO < >

Impairment (SUB AB)

1. <a> <b>
2. < >
3. <a> <b>
4. < >

Impairment (PHO)

1. < > home
2. < > school
3. < > peers

Impairment (SOCIAL PHO)

1. < > home
2. < > school
3. < > peers

Criteria (SUB AB)

   If any use (Q1–4) and any
  impairment (1–4), then criteria
     met SUB AB < >

Type(s) _____
_____
_____
_____

Type(s) (PHO)

Animal   < >
Natural Environment   < >
Blood–Injection–Injury   < >
Situational   < >
Other _____   < >

SEP ANX	GEN ANX	OCD

1. <a> <b>
2. <a> <b>
3. < >
4. <a> <b>
5. <a> <b>
6. <a> <b>
7. <a> <b>
8. <a> <b>
	1. < > _____
	_____
	_____
	_____
	_____
	2. <a> <b>
	3. <a> <b> <c> <d> <e> <f>
		A. Compulsions
		   1. < > _____
		   2. <a> _____
		      <b>
		   3. < >
		
		B. Obsessions
		   1. <a> _____
		      <b> _____
		      <c> _____
		   2. <a> <b> <c>
		   3. < >
		
		C. Interference
		   1. <a> <b> <c>

Criteria
  If ≥3, then criteria met
    SEP ANX < >
	Criteria
	  If 1–3, then criteria met
	    GEN ANX < >
		Criteria
		  If A1, A2, & C,
		  then criteria met
		  Compulsions < >
		
		  If B1, B2, & C,
		  then criteria met
		  Obsessions < >
		
		  If Compulsions +
		  and/or Obsessions +,
		  then criteria met
		  OCD < >

Duration
1. _____ (years old)
2. < > _____ (years old)
3. < > _____ (weeks)
 	
  *DUR met for SEP ANX < >
	Duration
	1. _____ (years old)
	2. < > _____ (years old)
	3. < > _____ (months)
	
	  *DUR met for GEN ANX < >
		Duration
		1. _____ (years old)
		2. < > _____ (years old)
		    _____ (months)
		
		  *DUR met for OCD < >

Impairment 1. < > home 2. < > school 3. < > peers	**Impairment** 1. < > home 2. < > school 3. < > peers	**Impairment** 1. < > home 2. < > school 3. < > peers

STRESS (ASD/PTSD)	ANO	BUL

A. Exposure
  1. \<a> \<b> _____
  2. \<a> \<b> \<c> \<d> \<e>
  3. \< > _____
B. Dissociation
  1. \<a> \<b> \<c> \<d>
  2. \< >
  3. \< >
  4. \< >
  5. \< >
C. Reexperiencing
  1. \<a> \<b> \<c>
  2. \<a> \<b>
  3. \<a> \<b>
  4. \<a> \<b>
  5. \< >
D. Avoidance
  1. \<a> \<b>
  2. \<a> \<b> \<c>
  3. \< >
  4. \<a> \<b>
  5. \<a> \<b>
  6. \<a> \<b>
  7. \<a> \<b>
E. Hyperarousal
  1. \<a> \<b>
  2. \<a> \<b>
  3. \< >
  4. \< >
  5. \< >
	1. \<a> \<b>
	2. \<a>
	  ht: _____
	  wt: _____
	  \<b>
	  ht: _____
	  wt: _____
	3. \<a> \<b> \<c>
	4. \<a> \<b> \<c>
	5. \< >
		1. \< > _____
		_____
		2. \<a> \<b> \<c> \<d>
		3. \<a> \<b> \<c> \<d>
		4. \<a> \<b>

Criteria If A1 & A2, ≥3 in B, ≥1 in C, ≥3 in D, and ≥2 in E, then criteria met ASD \< > If A1 & A2, ≥1 in C, ≥3 in D, and ≥2 in E, then criteria met PTSD \< >	**Criteria** If 1–4 (&5 for pubescent girls), then criteria met ANO \< >	**Criteria** If 1–4, then criteria met BUL \< >

Duration
1. _____ (years old)
2. \< > _____ (years old)
3. a. \< > _____ (weeks)
  b. \< >
  c. \< > _____ (days)
4. \< > _____ (months)
    *DUR met for ASD \< >
    *DUR met for PTSD \< >
	Duration
	1. _____ (years old)
	2. \< > _____ (years old)
	3. \< > _____ (months)
	
	    *DUR met for ANO \< >
		Duration
		1. _____ (years old)
		2. \< > _____ (years old)
		3. a. \< > _____ (#/week)
		  b. \< > _____ (months)
		
		    *DUR met for BUL \< >

Impairment 1. \< > home 2. \< > school 3. \< > peers	**Impairment** 1. \< > home 2. \< > school 3. \< > peers	**Impairment** 1. \< > home 2. \< > school 3. \< > peers
Type (PTSD) Acute \< > Regular Onset \< > Chronic \< > Delayed Onset \< >		

DEP/DYS (MDD/DD)	DEP/DYS (MDD/DD)	MAN/HYPOMAN
A. Dysphoric Mood 　1. \<a> \<b> \<c> 　2. \<a> \<bi> \<bii> \<biii> 　　\<c> \<d> B. Loss of Interest 　1. \<a> \<b> 　2. \<a> \<b> \<c> C. Appetite Changes 　1. \<a> \<b> \<c> 　2. \<a> \<b> D. Sleep Changes 　　Bedtime: _____ 　　Wakeup: _____ 　1. \<a> \<b> \<c> 　2. \<a> \<b> E. Psychomotor Changes 　1. \<a> \<b> \<c> \<d> 　2. \<a> \<b> F. Low Energy 　1. \<a> \<b> \<c> \<d> G. Guilt 　1. \<a> \<b> \<c> \<d> 　2. \<a> \<b> H. Impaired Concentration 　1. \<a> \<b> \<c> \<d> \<e> 　2. \< > I. Hopelessness 　1. \<a> \<b> \<c> J. Morbid/Suicidal Thoughts 　1. \<a> \<b> 　2. \<a> \<b> \<c> \<d> \<e> _____ _____ _____ _____ _____		A. Elevated Mood 　1. \<a> _____ 　　\<b> _____ 　　\<c> _____ 　2. \< > _____ B. Other Symptoms 　1. \<a> _____ 　　\<b> 　2. \<a> \<b> \<c> _____ 　3. \<a> \<b> \<c> \<d> 　4. \<a> \<b> \<c> 　5. \< > 　6. \<a> \<b> \<c> \<d> \<e> 　7. \<a> \<b> \<c> \<d> C. Interference 　1. \< > 　2. \< >
	Criteria If A &/or B & ≥5 of A–H or J, then criteria met MDD \< > If A & ≥2 of C, D, F, G, H, or I, then criteria met DD \< >	**Criteria** If A1(a, b, & c) + ≥3 in B + ≥1 in C *or* A2 + ≥4 in B + ≥1 in C, then criteria met MAN \< > If A1(a, b, & c) + ≥3 in B + none in C *or* A2 + ≥4 in B + none in C, then criteria met HYPOMAN \< >
	Duration 1. _____ (years old) 2. \< > _____ (years old) 3. MDD \< > _____ (weeks) 　DD　\< > _____ (months) 　*DUR met for MDD \< > 　*DUR met for DD \< >	**Duration** 1. _____ (years old) 2. \< > _____ (years old) 3. MAN \< > _____ (weeks) 　HYPO \< > _____ (days) 　*DUR met for MAN \< > 　*DUR met for HYPOMAN \< >
	Impairment 1. \< > home 2. \< > school 3. \< > peers	**Impairment** 1. \< > home 2. \< > school 3. \< > peers

ENU	SCZ/PSY	STRESSORS

1. < >
 2. \<a> \<b>
 3. \<a> \<b>
	A. Psychotic Symptoms
	   1. \<a> \<b> \<c> \<d> \<e>
	   2. \<a> \<b> \<c> \<d> \<e> \<f>
	   3. < >
	   4. < >
	   5. < >
		A. Child Abuse/Neglect
		 1. \<a> \<b> \<c>
		 2. \<a> \<b> \<c> \<d>
		 3. \<a> \<b> \<c> \<d>
		 4. < >
		 5. < >

Criteria
   If 1, ≥1 in 2, 3a, and 3b,
     then criteria met
       ENU < >
	B. Interference
	   1. < >
	   2. < >
	   3. < >
		Duration
		 1. _____
		 2. < > _____
		 3. _____
		 4. _____
		 5. < >

Duration
 1. _____ (years old)
 2. < > _____ (years old)
 3. \<a> _____ (x/week)
    \<b> _____ (months)
 	
   *DUR met for ENU < >
	Criteria
	   If ≥2 in A and ≥1 in B,
	     then criteria met
	       SCZ < >
	
	   If ≥1 in A, then criteria met
	       PSY < >
		B. Other Stressors
		  1. \<a> \<b> \<c> \<d> \<e>
		  2. < >
		  3. \<a> \<b>
		  4. \<a> \<b> \<c>
		  5. \<a> \<b>
		  6. \<a> \<b>
		  7. \<a> _____
		      \<b>
		  8. \<a> \<b> \<c> \<d>
		  9. < > _____
		      _____
		      _____
		 10. < >
		 11. < > _____
		      _____
		      _____

Impairment
 1. < > home
 2. < > school
 3. < > peers
	Duration
	 1. _____ (years old)
	 2. < > _____ (years old)
	 3. < > _____ (months)
	
	   *DUR met for SCZ < >
	   *DUR met for PSY < >	

Type Nocturnal < > Diurnal < > Both < >		
ENC	**Impairment** 1. < > home 2. < > school 3. < > peers	
1. < > 2. < >		
Criteria If both 1 & 2, then criteria met ENC < >		

Duration
 1. _____ (years old)
 2. < > _____ (years old)
 3. \<a> _____ (x/month)
    \<b> _____ (months)
 	
   *DUR met for ENC < >		

Impairment 1. < > home 2. < > school 3. < > peers		

| ChIPS Scoring Form |
| Profile Sheet |

Child's Number: _____ Date: _____

Child's Name: _____ Time Started: _____

Date of Birth: _____ Age: _____ Time Ended: _____

Race: _____ Sex: _____ Interviewer: _____

Setting (circle one):   Inpatient,   Outpatient,   School,   Other Research Setting: _____

	Disorder	Symptoms	Diagnosis	Duration	Clinician's Diagnosis
ADHD	Attention-Deficit/Hyperactivity Disorder	<>	<>	<>	Axis I
	Type: Inattentive, Hyperactive–Impulsive, Combined				
ODD	Oppositional Defiant Disorder	<>	<>	<>	
CD	Conduct Disorder	<>	<>	<>	
	Onset: Childhood, Adolescent				
	Severity: Mild, Moderate, Severe				
SUBAB	Substance Abuse	<>	<>	<>	
	Substance(s): _____				
PHO	Specific Phobia	<>	<>	<>	Axis II
	Type: _____				
SOCPHO	Social Phobia	<>	<>	<>	
SEPANX	Separation Anxiety Disorder	<>	<>	<>	Axis III
GENANX	General Anxiety Disorder	<>	<>	<>	
OCD	Obsessive-Compulsive Disorder	<>	<>	<>	
PTSD	Posttraumatic Stress Disorder	<>	<>	<>	Axis IV
	Type: Acute, Chronic				
	Onset: Regular, Delayed				
ASD	Acute Stress Disorder	<>	<>	<>	
ANO	Anorexia	<>	<>	<>	Axis V
BUL	Bulimia	<>	<>	<>	current:
DEP	Major Depressive Disorder	<>	<>	<>	past year:
DYS	Dysthymic Disorder	<>	<>	<>	
MAN	Mania	<>	<>	<>	
HYPOMAN	Hypomania	<>	<>	<>	
ENU	Enuresis	<>	<>	<>	
	Type: Nocturnal, Diurnal, Both				
ENC	Encopresis	<>	<>	<>	
SCZ	Schizophrenia	<>	<>	<>	
PSY	Psychosis	<>	<>	<>	

Psychosocial Stressors:

Other Stressors:

Behavioral Observations

Appearance: Affect:

Effort: Level of Activity:

Unusual Behaviors:

Presenting Problem

Home

1.

2.

School

1.

2.

3.

4.

5.

Peers/Work

1.

2.

3.

4.

5.

Medication

Type:

Dosage:

ADHD	ODD	CD

A. Inattention
  1. \<a> \<b>
  2. \< >
  3. \<a> \<b>
  4. \<a> \<b> \<c>
  5. \< >
  6. \< >
  7. \< >
  8. \<a> \<b>
  9. \<a> \<b>
 	
B. Hyperactivity–Impulsivity
  1. \<a> \<b>
  2. \<a> \<b>
  3. \< >
  4. \<a> \<b>
  5. \< >
  6. \<a> \<b>
  7. \< >
  8. \<a> \<b>
  9. \<a> \<b> \<c>
	1. \<a> \<b>
	2. \<a> \<b>
	3. \<a> \<b> \<c> \<d>
	4. \< >
	5. \<a> \<b>
	6. \< >
	7. \< >
	8. \< >
		1. \< >
		2. \<a> \<b>
		3. \< >
		4. \< >
		5. \< >
		6. \< >
		7. \<a> \<b>
		8. \<a> \<b>
		9. \< >
		10. \<a> \<b>
		11. \< >
		12. \< >
		13. \< >
		14. \< >
		15. \<a> \<b>

Criteria If ≥6 in *A only*, then criteria met Inattentive \< > If ≥6 in *B only*, then criteria met Hyperactive–Impulsive \< > If ≥6 in A *and* ≥6 in B, then criteria met Combined \< >	**Criteria** If ≥4, then criteria met ODD \< >	**Criteria** If ≥3, then criteria met CD \< >

Duration
1. _____ (years old)
2. \< > _____ (years old)
3. \< > _____ (months)
 	
  * DUR met for ADHD \< >
	Duration
	1. _____ (years old)
	2. \< > _____ (years old)
	3. \< > _____ (months)
	
	  * DUR met for ODD \< >
		Duration
		1. _____ (years old)
		2. \< > _____ (years old)
		3. \< > _____ (months)
		
		  * DUR met for CD \< >

Impairment 1. \< > home 2. \< > school 3. \< > peers	**Impairment** 1. \< > home 2. \< > school 3. \< > peers	**Impairment** 1. \< > home 2. \< > school 3. \< > peers
		Type Childhood Onset \< > Adolescent Onset \< > Mild \< > Moderate \< > Severe \< >

SUB AB	PHO	SOCIAL PHO

1. < >
    <a>_____
    <b>_____
    <c>_____
 	
    _____
2. < > _____
3. < > _____
4. < > _____
	1. _____
	   _____
	   _____
	2. <a> <b>
	3. <a> <b>
	4. <ai> <aii> <aiii> <aiv> <b>
	5. <a> <b>
		1. <a> <b>
		2. < >
		3. <a> <b>
		4. <ai> <aii> <aiii> <aiv> <b>
		5. < >

SUB AB	PHO	SOCIAL PHO

Duration
1. _____ (years old)
2. < > _____ (years old)
    _____ (months)
 	
  * DUR met for SUB AB < >
	Criteria
	  If 1–4, then criteria met
	      PHO < >
		Criteria
		  If 1–4, then criteria met
		  SOCIAL PHO < >

	Duration 1. _____ (years old) 2. < > _____ (years old) 3. < > _____ (months) * DUR met for PHO < >	**Duration** 1. _____ (years old) 2. < > _____ (years old) 3. < > _____ (months) *DUR met for SOCIAL PHO < >

SUB AB	PHO	SOCIAL PHO
Impairment 1. <a> <b> 2. < > 3. <a> <b> 4. < >	**Impairment** 1. < > home 2. < > school 3. < > peers	**Impairment** 1. < > home 2. < > school 3. < > peers

SUB AB	PHO	SOCIAL PHO

Criteria
  If any use (Q1–4) and any
  impairment (1–4), then criteria
    met SUB AB < >
 	
Type(s) _____
_____
_____
_____
	Type(s)
	Animal < >
	Natural Environment < >
	Blood–Injection–Injury < >
	Situational < >
	Other _____ < >	

SEP ANX	GEN ANX	OCD
1. <a> <b> 2. <a> <b> 3. < > 4. <a> <b> 5. <a> <b> 6. <a> <b> 7. <a> <b> 8. <a> <b>	1. < > _____ _____ _____ _____ _____ 2. <a> <b> 3. <a> <b> <c> <d> <e> <f>	A. Compulsions 　　1. < > _____ 　　2. <a> _____ 　　　　<b> 　　3. < > B. Obsessions 　　1. <a> _____ 　　　　<b> _____ 　　　　<c> _____ 　　2. <a> <b> <c> 　　3. < > C. Interference 　　1. <a> <b> <c>
Criteria 　If ≥3, then criteria met 　　SEP ANX < >	**Criteria** 　If 1–3, then criteria met 　　GEN ANX < >	**Criteria** 　If A1, A2, & C, 　then criteria met 　Compulsions < > 　If B1, B2, & C, 　then criteria met 　Obsessions < > 　If Compulsions + 　and/or Obsessions +, 　then criteria met 　　OCD < >
Duration 1. _____ (years old) 2. < > _____ (years old) 3. < > _____ (weeks) 　*DUR met for SEP ANX < >	**Duration** 1. _____ (years old) 2. < > _____ (years old) 3. < > _____ (months) 　*DUR met for GEN ANX < >	**Duration** 1. _____ (years old) 2. < > _____ (years old) 　　_____ (months) 　*DUR met for OCD < >
Impairment 1. < > home 2. < > school 3. < > peers	**Impairment** 1. < > home 2. < > school 3. < > peers	**Impairment** 1. < > home 2. < > school 3. < > peers

STRESS (ASD/PTSD)	ANO	BUL

A. Exposure
  1. \<a> \<b> _____
  2. \<a> \<b> \<c> \<d> \<e>
  3. \< > _____
B. Dissociation
  1. \<a> \<b> \<c> \<d>
  2. \< >
  3. \< >
  4. \< >
  5. \< >
C. Reexperiencing
  1. \<a> \<b> \<c>
  2. \<a> \<b>
  3. \<a> \<b>
  4. \<a> \<b>
  5. \< >
D. Avoidance
  1. \<a> \<b>
  2. \<a> \<b> \<c>
  3. \< >
  4. \<a> \<b>
  5. \<a> \<b>
  6. \<a> \<b>
  7. \<a> \<b>
E. Hyperarousal
  1. \<a> \<b>
  2. \<a> \<b>
  3. \< >
  4. \< >
  5. \< >
	1. \<a> \<b>
	2. \<a>
	  ht: _____
	  wt: _____
	  \<b>
	  ht: _____
	  wt: _____
	3. \<a> \<b> \<c>
	4. \<a> \<b> \<c>
	5. \< >
		1. \< > _____
		  _____
		2. \<a> \<b> \<c> \<d>
		3. \<a> \<b> \<c> \<d>
		4. \<a> \<b>

Criteria If A1 *&* A2, ≥3 in B, ≥1 in C, ≥3 in D, and ≥2 in E, then criteria met ASD \< > If A1 *&* A2, ≥1 in C, ≥3 in D, and ≥2 in E, then criteria met PTSD \< >	**Criteria** If 1–4 (&5 for pubescent girls), then criteria met ANO \< >	**Criteria** If 1–4, then criteria met BUL \< >

Duration
1. _____ (years old)
2. \< > _____ (years old)
3. a. \< > _____ (weeks)
   b. \< >
   c. \< > _____ (days)
4. \< > _____ (months)
     *DUR met for ASD \< >
     *DUR met for PTSD \< >
	Duration
	1. _____ (years old)
	2. \< > _____ (years old)
	3. \< > _____ (months)
	
	   *DUR met for ANO \< >
		Duration
		1. _____ (years old)
		2. \< > _____ (years old)
		3. a. \< > _____ (#/week)
		   b. \< > _____ (months)
		
		   *DUR met for BUL \< >

Impairment 1. \< > home 2. \< > school 3. \< > peers	**Impairment** 1. \< > home 2. \< > school 3. \< > peers	**Impairment** 1. \< > home 2. \< > school 3. \< > peers
Type (PTSD) Acute \< > Regular Onset \< > Chronic \< > Delayed Onset \< >		

DEP/DYS (MDD/DD)	DEP/DYS (MDD/DD)	MAN/HYPOMAN

A. Dysphoric Mood
 1. <a> <b> <c>
 2. <a> <bi> <bii> <biii>
  <c> <d>
 	
B. Loss of Interest
 1. <a> <b>
 2. <a> <b> <c>
 	
C. Appetite Changes
 1. <a> <b> <c>
 2. <a> <b>
 	
D. Sleep Changes
  Bedtime: _____
  Wakeup: _____
 1. <a> <b> <c>
 2. <a> <b>
 	
E. Psychomotor Changes
 1. <a> <b> <c> <d>
 2. <a> <b>
 	
F. Low Energy
 1. <a> <b> <c> <d>
 	
G. Guilt
 1. <a> <b> <c> <d>
 2. <a> <b>
 	
H. Impaired Concentration
 1. <a> <b> <c> <d> <e>
 2. < >
 	
I. Hopelessness
 1. <a> <b> <c>
 	
J. Morbid/Suicidal Thoughts
 1. <a> <b>
 2. <a> <b> <c> <d> <e>
 	
_____
_____
_____
_____
_____
		A. Elevated Mood
		 1. <a> _____
		  <b> _____
		  <c> _____
		 2. < > _____
		
		B. Other Symptoms
		 1. <a> _____
		  <b>
		 2. <a> <b> <c> _____
		 3. <a> <b> <c> <d>
		 4. <a> <b> <c>
		 5. < >
		 6. <a> <b> <c> <d> <e>
		 7. <a> <b> <c> <d>
		
		C. Interference
		 1. < >
		 2. < >

	Criteria If A &/or B & ≥5 of A–H or J, then criteria met MDD < > If A & ≥2 of C, D, F, G, H, or I, then criteria met DD < >	**Criteria** If A1(a, b, & c) + ≥3 in B + ≥1 in C *or* A2 + ≥4 in B + ≥1 in C, then criteria met MAN < > If A1(a, b, & c) + ≥3 in B + none in C *or* A2 + ≥4 in B + none in C, then criteria met HYPOMAN < >

	Duration
	1. _____ (years old)
	2. < > _____ (years old)
	3. MDD < > _____ (weeks)
	  DD < > _____ (months)
	
	*DUR met for MDD < >
	*DUR met for DD < >
		Duration
		1. _____ (years old)
		2. < > _____ (years old)
		3. MAN < > _____ (weeks)
		  HYPO < > _____ (days)
		
		*DUR met for MAN < >
		*DUR met for HYPOMAN < >

	Impairment 1. < > home 2. < > school 3. < > peers	**Impairment** 1. < > home 2. < > school 3. < > peers

ENU	SCZ/PSY	STRESSORS
1. < >	A. Psychotic Symptoms	A. Child Abuse/Neglect
2. <a> <b>	1. <a> <b> <c> <d> <e>	1. <a> <b> <c>
3. <a> <b>	2. <a> <b> <c> <d> <e> <f>	2. <a> <b> <c> <d>
	3. < >	3. <a> <b> <c> <d>
Criteria	4. < >	4. < >
If 1, ≥1 in 2, 3a, and 3b,	5. < >	5. < >
then criteria met		
ENU < >	B. Interference	**Duration**
	1. < >	1. _____
Duration	2. < >	2. < > _____
1. _____ (years old)	3. < >	3. _____
2. < > _____ (years old)		4. _____
3. <a> _____ (x/week)	**Criteria**	5. < >
<b> _____ (months)	If ≥2 in A and ≥1 in B,	
	then criteria met	B. Other Stressors
*DUR met for ENU < >	SCZ < >	1. <a> <b> <c> <d> <e>
		2. < >
Impairment	If ≥1 in A, then criteria met	3. <a> <b>
1. < > home	PSY < >	4. <a> <b> <c>
2. < > school		5. <a> <b>
3. < > peers		6. <a> <b>
	Duration	7. <a> _____
Type	1. _____ (years old)	<b>
Nocturnal < >	2. < > _____ (years old)	8. <a> <b> <c> <d>
Diurnal < >	3. < > _____ (months)	9. < > _____
Both < >		_____
	*DUR met for SCZ < >	_____
ENC	*DUR met for PSY < >	10. < >
		11. < > _____
1. < >	**Impairment**	_____
2. < >	1. < > home	_____
	2. < > school	_____
Criteria	3. < > peers	
If both 1 & 2, then criteria met		
ENC < >		
Duration		
1. _____ (years old)		
2. < > _____ (years old)		
3. <a> _____ (x/month)		
<b> _____ (months)		
*DUR met for ENC < >		
Impairment		
1. < > home		
2. < > school		
3. < > peers		

ChIPS Scoring Form
Profile Sheet

Child's Number: _____ Date: _____

Child's Name: _____ Time Started: _____

Date of Birth: _____ Age: _____ Time Ended: _____

Race: _____ Sex: _____ Interviewer: _____

Setting (circle one): Inpatient, Outpatient, School, Other Research Setting: _____

	Disorder	Symptoms	Diagnosis	Duration	Clinician's Diagnosis
ADHD	**Attention-Deficit/Hyperactivity Disorder** *Type:* Inattentive, Hyperactive–Impulsive, Combined	<>	<>	<>	**Axis I**
ODD	**Oppositional Defiant Disorder**	<>	<>	<>	
CD	**Conduct Disorder** *Onset:* Childhood, Adolescent *Severity:* Mild, Moderate, Severe	<>	<>	<>	
SUBAB	**Substance Abuse** *Substance(s):* _____	<>	<>	<>	
PHO	**Specific Phobia** *Type:* _____	<>	<>	<>	**Axis II**
SOCPHO	**Social Phobia**	<>	<>	<>	
SEPANX	**Separation Anxiety Disorder**	<>	<>	<>	**Axis III**
GENANX	**General Anxiety Disorder**	<>	<>	<>	
OCD	**Obsessive-Compulsive Disorder**	<>	<>	<>	
PTSD	**Posttraumatic Stress Disorder** *Type:* Acute, Chronic *Onset:* Regular, Delayed	<>	<>	<>	**Axis IV**
ASD	**Acute Stress Disorder**	<>	<>	<>	
ANO	**Anorexia**	<>	<>	<>	**Axis V**
BUL	**Bulimia**	<>	<>	<>	current:
DEP	**Major Depressive Disorder**	<>	<>	<>	past year:
DYS	**Dysthymic Disorder**	<>	<>	<>	
MAN	**Mania**	<>	<>	<>	
HYPOMAN	**Hypomania**	<>	<>	<>	
ENU	**Enuresis** *Type:* Nocturnal, Diurnal, Both	<>	<>	<>	
ENC	**Encopresis**	<>	<>	<>	
SCZ	**Schizophrenia**	<>	<>	<>	
PSY	**Psychosis**	<>	<>	<>	

Psychosocial Stressors:

Other Stressors:

Behavioral Observations

Appearance: Affect:

Effort: Level of Activity:

Unusual Behaviors:

Presenting Problem

Home

1.

2.

School

1.

2.

3.

4.

5.

Peers/Work

1.

2.

3.

4.

5.

Medication

Type:

Dosage:

ChIPS Scoring Form

ADHD	ODD	CD

A. Inattention
  1. <a> <b>
  2. < >
  3. <a> <b>
  4. <a> <b> <c>
  5. < >
  6. < >
  7. < >
  8. <a> <b>
  9. <a> <b>
 	
B. Hyperactivity–Impulsivity
  1. <a> <b>
  2. <a> <b>
  3. < >
  4. <a> <b>
  5. < >
  6. <a> <b>
  7. < >
  8. <a> <b>
  9. <a> <b> <c>
	1. <a> <b>
	2. <a> <b>
	3. <a> <b> <c> <d>
	4. < >
	5. <a> <b>
	6. < >
	7. < >
	8. < >
		1. < >
		2. <a> <b>
		3. < >
		4. < >
		5. < >
		6. < >
		7. <a> <b>
		8. <a> <b>
		9. < >
		10. <a> <b>
		11. < >
		12. < >
		13. < >
		14. < >
		15. <a> <b>

Criteria If ≥6 in *A only*, then criteria met Inattentive < > If ≥6 in *B only*, then criteria met Hyperactive–Impulsive < > If ≥6 in A *and* ≥6 in B, then criteria met Combined < >	**Criteria** If ≥4, then criteria met ODD < >	**Criteria** If ≥3, then criteria met CD < >

Duration
1. _____ (years old)
2. < > _____ (years old)
3. < > _____ (months)
 	
  * DUR met for ADHD < >
	Duration
	1. _____ (years old)
	2. < > _____ (years old)
	3. < > _____ (months)
	
	  * DUR met for ODD < >
		Duration
		1. _____ (years old)
		2. < > _____ (years old)
		3. < > _____ (months)
		
		  * DUR met for CD < >

Impairment 1. < > home 2. < > school 3. < > peers	**Impairment** 1. < > home 2. < > school 3. < > peers	**Impairment** 1. < > home 2. < > school 3. < > peers
		Type Childhood Onset < > Adolescent Onset < > Mild < > Moderate < > Severe < >

SUB AB	PHO	SOCIAL PHO

1. < >
    <a>_____
    <b>_____
    <c>_____
 	
    _____
2. < > _____
3. < > _____
4. < > _____
	1. _____
	    _____
	    _____
	2. <a> <b>
	3. <a> <b>
	4. <ai> <aii> <aiii> <aiv> <b>
	5. <a> <b>
		1. <a> <b>
		2. < >
		3. <a> <b>
		4. <ai> <aii> <aiii> <aiv> <b>
		5. < >

Duration
1. _____ (years old)
2. < > _____ (years old)
    _____ (months)
 	
  * DUR met for SUB AB < >
	Criteria
	  If 1–4, then criteria met
	    PHO < >
		Criteria
		  If 1–4, then criteria met
		    SOCIAL PHO < >

	Duration
	1. _____ (years old)
	2. < > _____ (years old)
	3. < > _____ (months)
	
	  * DUR met for PHO < >
		Duration
		1. _____ (years old)
		2. < > _____ (years old)
		3. < > _____ (months)
		
		  *DUR met for SOCIAL PHO < >

Impairment 1. <a> <b> 2. < > 3. <a> <b> 4. < >	**Impairment** 1. < > home 2. < > school 3. < > peers	**Impairment** 1. < > home 2. < > school 3. < > peers

Criteria
  If any use (Q1–4) and any
  impairment (1–4), then criteria
    met SUB AB < >
 	
Type(s) _____
  _____
  _____
  _____
	Type(s)
	Animal < >
	Natural Environment < >
	Blood–Injection–Injury < >
	Situational < >
	Other _____ < >	

SEP ANX	GEN ANX	OCD

1. \<a\> \<b\>
2. \<a\> \<b\>
3. \< \>
4. \<a\> \<b\>
5. \<a\> \<b\>
6. \<a\> \<b\>
7. \<a\> \<b\>
8. \<a\> \<b\>
	1. \< \> _____
	_____
	_____
	_____
	_____
	2. \<a\> \<b\>
	3. \<a\> \<b\> \<c\> \<d\> \<e\> \<f\>
		A. Compulsions
		  1. \< \> _____
		  2. \<a\> _____
		    \<b\>
		  3. \< \>
		
		B. Obsessions
		  1. \<a\> _____
		    \<b\> _____
		    \<c\> _____
		  2. \<a\> \<b\> \<c\>
		  3. \< \>
		
		C. Interference
		  1. \<a\> \<b\> \<c\>

Criteria If ≥3, then criteria met SEP ANX \< \>	**Criteria** If 1–3, then criteria met GEN ANX \< \>	**Criteria** If A1, A2, & C, then criteria met Compulsions \< \> If B1, B2, & C, then criteria met Obsessions \< \> If Compulsions + and/or Obsessions +, then criteria met OCD \< \>
Duration 1. _____ (years old) 2. \< \> _____ (years old) 3. \< \> _____ (weeks) *DUR met for SEP ANX \< \>	**Duration** 1. _____ (years old) 2. \< \> _____ (years old) 3. \< \> _____ (months) *DUR met for GEN ANX \< \>	**Duration** 1. _____ (years old) 2. \< \> _____ (years old) _____ (months) *DUR met for OCD \< \>
Impairment 1. \< \> home 2. \< \> school 3. \< \> peers	**Impairment** 1. \< \> home 2. \< \> school 3. \< \> peers	**Impairment** 1. \< \> home 2. \< \> school 3. \< \> peers

STRESS (ASD/PTSD)	ANO	BUL

A. Exposure
   1. \<a> \<b> _____
   2. \<a> \<b> \<c> \<d> \<e>
   3. \< > _____
B. Dissociation
   1. \<a> \<b> \<c> \<d>
   2. \< >
   3. \< >
   4. \< >
   5. \< >
C. Reexperiencing
   1. \<a> \<b> \<c>
   2. \<a> \<b>
   3. \<a> \<b>
   4. \<a> \<b>
   5. \< >
D. Avoidance
   1. \<a> \<b>
   2. \<a> \<b> \<c>
   3. \< >
   4. \<a> \<b>
   5. \<a> \<b>
   6. \<a> \<b>
   7. \<a> \<b>
E. Hyperarousal
   1. \<a> \<b>
   2. \<a> \<b>
   3. \< >
   4. \< >
   5. \< >
	1. \<a> \<b>
	2. \<a>
	   ht: _____
	   wt: _____
	  \<b>
	   ht: _____
	   wt: _____
	3. \<a> \<b> \<c>
	4. \<a> \<b> \<c>
	5. \< >
		1. \< > _____
		_____
		
		2. \<a> \<b> \<c> \<d>
		3. \<a> \<b> \<c> \<d>
		4. \<a> \<b>

Criteria If A1 & A2, ≥3 in B, ≥1 in C, ≥3 in D, and ≥2 in E, then criteria met ASD \< > If A1 & A2, ≥1 in C, ≥3 in D, and ≥2 in E, then criteria met PTSD \< >	**Criteria** If 1–4 (&5 for pubescent girls), then criteria met ANO \< >	**Criteria** If 1–4, then criteria met BUL \< >

Duration
1. _____ (years old)
2. \< > _____ (years old)
3. a. \< > _____ (weeks)
   b. \< >
   c. \< > _____ (days)
4. \< > _____ (months)
     *DUR met for ASD \< >
     *DUR met for PTSD \< >
	Duration
	1. _____ (years old)
	2. \< > _____ (years old)
	3. \< > _____ (months)
	
	    *DUR met for ANO \< >
		Duration
		1. _____ (years old)
		2. \< > _____ (years old)
		3. a. \< > _____ (#/week)
		   b. \< > _____ (months)
		
		    *DUR met for BUL \< >

Impairment 1. \< > home 2. \< > school 3. \< > peers	**Impairment** 1. \< > home 2. \< > school 3. \< > peers	**Impairment** 1. \< > home 2. \< > school 3. \< > peers
Type (PTSD) Acute \< > Regular Onset \< > Chronic \< > Delayed Onset \< >		

DEP/DYS (MDD/DD)	DEP/DYS (MDD/DD)	MAN/HYPOMAN

A. Dysphoric Mood
  1. \<a\> \<b\> \<c\>
  2. \<a\> \<bi\> \<bii\> \<biii\>
     \<c\> \<d\>
 	
B. Loss of Interest
  1. \<a\> \<b\>
  2. \<a\> \<b\> \<c\>
 	
C. Appetite Changes
  1. \<a\> \<b\> \<c\>
  2. \<a\> \<b\>
 	
D. Sleep Changes
     Bedtime: _____
     Wakeup: _____
  1. \<a\> \<b\> \<c\>
  2. \<a\> \<b\>
 	
E. Psychomotor Changes
  1. \<a\> \<b\> \<c\> \<d\>
  2. \<a\> \<b\>
 	
F. Low Energy
  1. \<a\> \<b\> \<c\> \<d\>
 	
G. Guilt
  1. \<a\> \<b\> \<c\> \<d\>
  2. \<a\> \<b\>
 	
H. Impaired Concentration
  1. \<a\> \<b\> \<c\> \<d\> \<e\>
  2. \< \>
 	
I. Hopelessness
  1. \<a\> \<b\> \<c\>
 	
J. Morbid/Suicidal Thoughts
  1. \<a\> \<b\>
  2. \<a\> \<b\> \<c\> \<d\> \<e\>
 	
_____
_____
_____
_____
_____
		A. Elevated Mood
		  1. \<a\> _____
		     \<b\> _____
		     \<c\> _____
		  2. \< \> _____
		
		B. Other Symptoms
		  1. \<a\> _____
		     \<b\>
		  2. \<a\> \<b\> \<c\> _____
		  3. \<a\> \<b\> \<c\> \<d\>
		  4. \<a\> \<b\> \<c\>
		  5. \< \>
		  6. \<a\> \<b\> \<c\> \<d\> \<e\>
		  7. \<a\> \<b\> \<c\> \<d\>
		
		C. Interference
		  1. \< \>
		  2. \< \>

	Criteria
	  If A &/or B & ≥5 of A–H or J,
	  then criteria met
	  MDD \< \>
	
	  If A & ≥2 of C, D, F, G, H, or I,
	  then criteria met
	  DD \< \>
		Criteria
		  If A1(a, b, & c) + ≥3 in B + ≥1 in C
		  or
		  A2 + ≥4 in B + ≥1 in C,
		  then criteria met
		  MAN \< \>
		
		  If A1(a, b, & c) + ≥3 in B +
		  none in C
		  or
		  A2 + ≥4 in B + none in C,
		  then criteria met
		  HYPOMAN \< \>

	Duration
	  1. _____ (years old)
	  2. \< \> _____ (years old)
	  3. MDD \< \> _____ (weeks)
	     DD \< \> _____ (months)
	
	  *DUR met for MDD \< \>
	  *DUR met for DD \< \>
		Duration
		  1. _____ (years old)
		  2. \< \> _____ (years old)
		  3. MAN \< \> _____ (weeks)
		     HYPO \< \> _____ (days)
		
		  *DUR met for MAN \< \>
		  *DUR met for HYPOMAN \< \>

	Impairment
	  1. \< \> home
	  2. \< \> school
	  3. \< \> peers
		Impairment
		  1. \< \> home
		  2. \< \> school
		  3. \< \> peers

ENU	SCZ/PSY	STRESSORS

1. < >
 2. <a> <b>
 3. <a> <b>
	A. Psychotic Symptoms
	   1. <a> <b> <c> <d> <e>
	   2. <a> <b> <c> <d> <e> <f>
	   3. < >
	   4. < >
	   5. < >
		A. Child Abuse/Neglect
		   1. <a> <b> <c>
		   2. <a> <b> <c> <d>
		   3. <a> <b> <c> <d>
		   4. < >
		   5. < >

Criteria
   If 1, ≥1 in 2, 3a, and 3b,
   then criteria met
     ENU < >
	B. Interference
	   1. < >
	   2. < >
	   3. < >
		Duration
		 1. _____
		 2. < > _____
		 3. _____
		 4. _____
		 5. < >

Duration
 1. _____ (years old)
 2. < > _____ (years old)
 3. <a> _____ (x/week)
    <b> _____ (months)
 	
   *DUR met for ENU < >
	Criteria
	   If ≥2 in A and ≥1 in B,
	   then criteria met
	     SCZ < >
	
	   If ≥1 in A, then criteria met
	     PSY < >
		B. Other Stressors
		   1. <a> <b> <c> <d> <e>
		   2. < >
		   3. <a> <b>
		   4. <a> <b> <c>
		   5. <a> <b>
		   6. <a> <b>
		   7. <a> _____
		      <b>
		   8. <a> <b> <c> <d>
		   9. < > _____

Impairment 1. < > home 2. < > school 3. < > peers		

Type
 Nocturnal   < >
 Diurnal   < >
 Both   < >
	Duration
	 1. _____ (years old)
	 2. < > _____ (years old)
	 3. < > _____ (months)
	
	   *DUR met for SCZ < >
	   *DUR met for PSY < >
		_____
		   10. < >
		   11. < > _____
		       _____
		       _____

ENC		
1. < > 2. < >	**Impairment** 1. < > home 2. < > school 3. < > peers	
Criteria If both 1 & 2, then criteria met ENC < >		
Duration 1. _____ (years old) 2. < > _____ (years old) 3. <a> _____ (x/month) <b> _____ (months) *DUR met for ENC < >		
Impairment 1. < > home 2. < > school 3. < > peers		

ChIPS Scoring Form
Profile Sheet

Child's Number: _____ Date: _____

Child's Name: _____ Time Started: _____

Date of Birth: _____ Age: _____ Time Ended: _____

Race: _____ Sex: _____ Interviewer: _____

Setting (circle one):   Inpatient,   Outpatient,   School,   Other Research Setting: _____

	Disorder	Symptoms	Diagnosis	Duration	Clinician's Diagnosis
ADHD	Attention-Deficit/Hyperactivity Disorder	<>	<>	<>	Axis I
	Type: Inattentive, Hyperactive–Impulsive, Combined				
ODD	Oppositional Defiant Disorder	<>	<>	<>	
CD	Conduct Disorder	<>	<>	<>	
	Onset: Childhood, Adolescent				
	Severity: Mild, Moderate, Severe				
SUBAB	Substance Abuse	<>	<>	<>	
	Substance(s): _____				
PHO	Specific Phobia	<>	<>	<>	Axis II
	Type: _____				
SOCPHO	Social Phobia	<>	<>	<>	
SEPANX	Separation Anxiety Disorder	<>	<>	<>	Axis III
GENANX	General Anxiety Disorder	<>	<>	<>	
OCD	Obsessive-Compulsive Disorder	<>	<>	<>	
PTSD	Posttraumatic Stress Disorder	<>	<>	<>	Axis IV
	Type: Acute, Chronic				
	Onset: Regular, Delayed				
ASD	Acute Stress Disorder	<>	<>	<>	
ANO	Anorexia	<>	<>	<>	Axis V
BUL	Bulimia	<>	<>	<>	current:
DEP	Major Depressive Disorder	<>	<>	<>	past year:
DYS	Dysthymic Disorder	<>	<>	<>	
MAN	Mania	<>	<>	<>	
HYPOMAN	Hypomania	<>	<>	<>	
ENU	Enuresis	<>	<>	<>	
	Type: Nocturnal, Diurnal, Both				
ENC	Encopresis	<>	<>	<>	
SCZ	Schizophrenia	<>	<>	<>	
PSY	Psychosis	<>	<>	<>	

Psychosocial Stressors:

Other Stressors:

Behavioral Observations

Appearance: Affect:

Effort: Level of Activity:

Unusual Behaviors:

Presenting Problem

Home

1.

2.

School

1.

2.

3.

4.

5.

Peers/Work

1.

2.

3.

4.

5.

Medication

Type:

Dosage:

Child's Name: _____

Date: _____

ADHD	ODD	CD

A. Inattention
  1. \<a> \<b>
  2. \< >
  3. \<a> \<b>
  4. \<a> \<b> \<c>
  5. \< >
  6. \< >
  7. \< >
  8. \<a> \<b>
  9. \<a> \<b>
 	
B. Hyperactivity–Impulsivity
  1. \<a> \<b>
  2. \<a> \<b>
  3. \< >
  4. \<a> \<b>
  5. \< >
  6. \<a> \<b>
  7. \< >
  8. \<a> \<b>
  9. \<a> \<b> \<c>
	1. \<a> \<b>
	2. \<a> \<b>
	3. \<a> \<b> \<c> \<d>
	4. \< >
	5. \<a> \<b>
	6. \< >
	7. \< >
	8. \< >
		1. \< >
		2. \<a> \<b>
		3. \< >
		4. \< >
		5. \< >
		6. \< >
		7. \<a> \<b>
		8. \<a> \<b>
		9. \< >
		10. \<a> \<b>
		11. \< >
		12. \< >
		13. \< >
		14. \< >
		15. \<a> \<b>

Criteria If ≥6 in *A only*, then criteria met Inattentive \< > If ≥6 in *B only*, then criteria met Hyperactive–Impulsive \< > If ≥6 in A *and* ≥6 in B, then criteria met Combined \< >	**Criteria** If ≥4, then criteria met ODD \< >	**Criteria** If ≥3, then criteria met CD \< >

Duration
1. _____ (years old)
2. \< > _____ (years old)
3. \< > _____ (months)
 	
  * DUR met for ADHD \< >
	Duration
	1. _____ (years old)
	2. \< > _____ (years old)
	3. \< > _____ (months)
	
	  * DUR met for ODD \< >
		Duration
		1. _____ (years old)
		2. \< > _____ (years old)
		3. \< > _____ (months)
		
		  * DUR met for CD \< >

Impairment 1. \< > home 2. \< > school 3. \< > peers	**Impairment** 1. \< > home 2. \< > school 3. \< > peers	**Impairment** 1. \< > home 2. \< > school 3. \< > peers
		Type Childhood Onset \< > Adolescent Onset \< > Mild \< > Moderate \< > Severe \< >

SUB AB	PHO	SOCIAL PHO

1. < >
    <a>_____
    <b>_____
    <c>_____
 	
    _____
2. < > _____
3. < > _____
4. < > _____
	1. _____
	   _____
	   _____
	2. <a> <b>
	3. <a> <b>
	4. <ai> <aii> <aiii> <aiv> <b>
	5. <a> <b>
		1. <a> <b>
		2. < >
		3. <a> <b>
		4. <ai> <aii> <aiii> <aiv> <b>
		5. < >

Duration
1. _____ (years old)
2. < > _____ (years old)
    _____ (months)
 	
  * DUR met for SUB AB < >
	Criteria
	  If 1–4, then criteria met
	      PHO < >
		Criteria
		  If 1–4, then criteria met
		    SOCIAL PHO < >

	Duration
	1. _____ (years old)
	2. < > _____ (years old)
	3. < > _____ (months)
	
	   * DUR met for PHO < >
		Duration
		1. _____ (years old)
		2. < > _____ (years old)
		3. < > _____ (months)
		
		  *DUR met for SOCIAL PHO < >

Impairment 1. <a> <b> 2. < > 3. <a> <b> 4. < >	**Impairment** 1. < > home 2. < > school 3. < > peers	**Impairment** 1. < > home 2. < > school 3. < > peers

Criteria
  If any use (Q1–4) and any
  impairment (1–4), then criteria
     met SUB AB < >
 	
Type(s) _____
_____
_____
_____
	Type(s)
	Animal < >
	Natural Environment < >
	Blood–Injection–Injury < >
	Situational < >
	Other _____ < >	

SEP ANX	GEN ANX	OCD

1. \<a\> \<b\>
2. \<a\> \<b\>
3. \< \>
4. \<a\> \<b\>
5. \<a\> \<b\>
6. \<a\> \<b\>
7. \<a\> \<b\>
8. \<a\> \<b\>
	1. \< \> _____
	    _____
	    _____
	    _____
	    _____
	2. \<a\> \<b\>
	3. \<a\> \<b\> \<c\> \<d\> \<e\> \<f\>
		A. Compulsions
		    1. \< \> _____
		    2. \<a\> _____
		        \<b\>
		    3. \< \>
		
		B. Obsessions
		    1. \<a\> _____
		        \<b\> _____
		        \<c\> _____
		    2. \<a\> \<b\> \<c\>
		    3. \< \>
		
		C. Interference
		    1. \<a\> \<b\> \<c\>

Criteria
    If ≥3, then criteria met
    SEP ANX \< \>
	Criteria
	    If 1–3, then criteria met
	    GEN ANX \< \>
		Criteria
		    If A1, A2, & C,
		    then criteria met
		    Compulsions \< \>
		
		    If B1, B2, & C,
		    then criteria met
		    Obsessions \< \>
		
		    If Compulsions +
		    and/or Obsessions +,
		    then criteria met
		    OCD \< \>

Duration
1. _____ (years old)
2. \< \> _____ (years old)
3. \< \> _____ (weeks)
 	
    *DUR met for SEP ANX \< \>
	Duration
	1. _____ (years old)
	2. \< \> _____ (years old)
	3. \< \> _____ (months)
	
	    *DUR met for GEN ANX \< \>
		Duration
		1. _____ (years old)
		2. \< \> _____ (years old)
		    _____ (months)
		
		    *DUR met for OCD \< \>

Impairment 1. \< \> home 2. \< \> school 3. \< \> peers	**Impairment** 1. \< \> home 2. \< \> school 3. \< \> peers	**Impairment** 1. \< \> home 2. \< \> school 3. \< \> peers

STRESS (ASD/PTSD)	ANO	BUL

A. Exposure
  1. \<a> \<b> _____
  2. \<a> \<b> \<c> \<d> \<e>
  3. \< > _____
B. Dissociation
  1. \<a> \<b> \<c> \<d>
  2. \< >
  3. \< >
  4. \< >
  5. \< >
C. Reexperiencing
  1. \<a> \<b> \<c>
  2. \<a> \<b>
  3. \<a> \<b>
  4. \<a> \<b>
  5. \< >
D. Avoidance
  1. \<a> \<b>
  2. \<a> \<b> \<c>
  3. \< >
  4. \<a> \<b>
  5. \<a> \<b>
  6. \<a> \<b>
  7. \<a> \<b>
E. Hyperarousal
  1. \<a> \<b>
  2. \<a> \<b>
  3. \< >
  4. \< >
  5. \< >
	1. \<a> \<b>
	2. \<a>
	  ht: _____
	  wt: _____
	 \<b>
	  ht: _____
	  wt: _____
	3. \<a> \<b> \<c>
	4. \<a> \<b> \<c>
	5. \< >
		1. \< > _____
		_____
		
		2. \<a> \<b> \<c> \<d>
		3. \<a> \<b> \<c> \<d>
		4. \<a> \<b>

Criteria If A1 & A2, ≥3 in B, ≥1 in C, ≥3 in D, and ≥2 in E, then criteria met ASD \< > If A1 & A2, ≥1 in C, ≥3 in D, and ≥2 in E, then criteria met PTSD \< >	**Criteria** If 1–4 (&5 for pubescent girls), then criteria met ANO \< >	**Criteria** If 1–4, then criteria met BUL \< >

Duration
1. _____ (years old)
2. \< > _____ (years old)
3. a. \< > _____ (weeks)
   b. \< >
   c. \< > _____ (days)
4. \< > _____ (months)
    *DUR met for ASD \< >
    *DUR met for PTSD \< >
	Duration
	1. _____ (years old)
	2. \< > _____ (years old)
	3. \< > _____ (months)
	
	   *DUR met for ANO \< >
		Duration
		1. _____ (years old)
		2. \< > _____ (years old)
		3. a. \< > _____ (#/week)
		   b. \< > _____ (months)
		
		   *DUR met for BUL \< >

Impairment 1. \< > home 2. \< > school 3. \< > peers	**Impairment** 1. \< > home 2. \< > school 3. \< > peers	**Impairment** 1. \< > home 2. \< > school 3. \< > peers
Type (PTSD) Acute \< > Regular Onset \< > Chronic \< > Delayed Onset \< >		

ChIPS Scoring Form

DEP/DYS (MDD/DD)	DEP/DYS (MDD/DD)	MAN/HYPOMAN

A. Dysphoric Mood
  1. \<a> \<b> \<c>
  2. \<a> \<bi> \<bii> \<biii>
     \<c> \<d>
 	
B. Loss of Interest
  1. \<a> \<b>
  2. \<a> \<b> \<c>
 	
C. Appetite Changes
  1. \<a> \<b> \<c>
  2. \<a> \<b>
 	
D. Sleep Changes
     Bedtime: _____
     Wakeup: _____
  1. \<a> \<b> \<c>
  2. \<a> \<b>
 	
E. Psychomotor Changes
  1. \<a> \<b> \<c> \<d>
  2. \<a> \<b>
 	
F. Low Energy
  1. \<a> \<b> \<c> \<d>
 	
G. Guilt
  1. \<a> \<b> \<c> \<d>
  2. \<a> \<b>
 	
H. Impaired Concentration
  1. \<a> \<b> \<c> \<d> \<e>
  2. \< >
 	
I. Hopelessness
  1. \<a> \<b> \<c>
 	
J. Morbid/Suicidal Thoughts
  1. \<a> \<b>
  2. \<a> \<b> \<c> \<d> \<e>
 	
_____
_____
_____
_____
_____
		A. Elevated Mood
		  1. \<a> _____
		     \<b> _____
		     \<c> _____
		  2. \< > _____
		
		B. Other Symptoms
		  1. \<a> _____
		     \<b>
		  2. \<a> \<b> \<c> _____
		  3. \<a> \<b> \<c> \<d>
		  4. \<a> \<b> \<c>
		  5. \< >
		  6. \<a> \<b> \<c> \<d> \<e>
		  7. \<a> \<b> \<c> \<d>
		
		C. Interference
		  1. \< >
		  2. \< >

	Criteria If A &/or B & ≥5 of A–H or J, then criteria met MDD \< > If A & ≥2 of C, D, F, G, H, or I, then criteria met DD \< >	**Criteria** If A1(a, b, & c) + ≥3 in B + ≥1 in C *or* A2 + ≥4 in B + ≥1 in C, then criteria met MAN \< > If A1(a, b, & c) + ≥3 in B + none in C *or* A2 + ≥4 in B + none in C, then criteria met HYPOMAN \< >

	Duration
	1. _____ (years old)
	2. \< > _____ (years old)
	3. MDD \< > _____ (weeks)
	   DD \< > _____ (months)
	
	  *DUR met for MDD \< >
	  *DUR met for DD \< >
		Duration
		1. _____ (years old)
		2. \< > _____ (years old)
		3. MAN \< > _____ (weeks)
		   HYPO \< > _____ (days)
		
		  *DUR met for MAN \< >
		  *DUR met for HYPOMAN \< >

	Impairment 1. \< > home 2. \< > school 3. \< > peers	**Impairment** 1. \< > home 2. \< > school 3. \< > peers

ENU	SCZ/PSY	STRESSORS

1. < >
 2. <a> <b>
 3. <a> <b>
 	
 Criteria
 If 1, ≥1 in 2, 3a, and 3b,
 then criteria met
 ENU < >
 	
 Duration
 1. _____ (years old)
 2. < > _____ (years old)
 3. <a> _____ (x/week)
    <b> _____ (months)
 	
   *DUR met for ENU < >
 	
 Impairment
 1. < > home
 2. < > school
 3. < > peers
 	
 Type
 Nocturnal   < >
 Diurnal   < >
 Both   < >
	A. Psychotic Symptoms
	    1. <a> <b> <c> <d> <e>
	    2. <a> <b> <c> <d> <e> <f>
	    3. < >
	    4. < >
	    5. < >
	
	 B. Interference
	    1. < >
	    2. < >
	    3. < >
	
	 Criteria
	 If ≥2 in A and ≥1 in B,
	 then criteria met
	 SCZ < >
	
	 If ≥1 in A, then criteria met
	 PSY < >
	
	 Duration
	 1. _____ (years old)
	 2. < > _____ (years old)
	 3. < > _____ (months)
	
	   *DUR met for SCZ < >
	   *DUR met for PSY < >
		A. Child Abuse/Neglect
		 1. <a> <b> <c>
		 2. <a> <b> <c> <d>
		 3. <a> <b> <c> <d>
		 4. < >
		 5. < >
		
		 Duration
		 1. _____
		 2. < > _____
		 3. _____
		 4. _____
		 5. < >

ENC (continued below ENU column)

1. < >
2. < >

Criteria
If both 1 & 2, then criteria met
ENC < >

Duration
1. _____ (years old)
2. < > _____ (years old)
3. <a> _____ (x/month)
   <b> _____ (months)

  *DUR met for ENC < >

Impairment
1. < > home
2. < > school
3. < > peers

Impairment (SCZ/PSY)
1. < > home
2. < > school
3. < > peers

B. Other Stressors
   1. <a> <b> <c> <d> <e>
   2. < >
   3. <a> <b>
   4. <a> <b> <c>
   5. <a> <b>
   6. <a> <b>
   7. <a> _____
       <b>
   8. <a> <b> <c> <d>
   9. < > _____
       _____
       _____
  10. < >
  11. < > _____
       _____
       _____

ChIPS Scoring Form
Profile Sheet

Child's Number: _____ Date: _____

Child's Name: _____ Time Started: _____

Date of Birth: _____ Age: _____ Time Ended: _____

Race: _____ Sex: _____ Interviewer: _____

Setting (circle one): Inpatient, Outpatient, School, Other Research Setting: _____

	Disorder	Symptoms	Diagnosis	Duration	Clinician's Diagnosis
ADHD	**Attention-Deficit/Hyperactivity Disorder**	<>	<>	<>	**Axis I**
	Type: Inattentive, Hyperactive–Impulsive, Combined				
ODD	**Oppositional Defiant Disorder**	<>	<>	<>	
CD	**Conduct Disorder**	<>	<>	<>	
	Onset: Childhood, Adolescent				
	Severity: Mild, Moderate, Severe				
SUBAB	**Substance Abuse**	<>	<>	<>	
	Substance(s): _____				
PHO	**Specific Phobia**	<>	<>	<>	**Axis II**
	Type: _____				
SOCPHO	**Social Phobia**	<>	<>	<>	
SEPANX	**Separation Anxiety Disorder**	<>	<>	<>	**Axis III**
GENANX	**General Anxiety Disorder**	<>	<>	<>	
OCD	**Obsessive-Compulsive Disorder**	<>	<>	<>	
PTSD	**Posttraumatic Stress Disorder**	<>	<>	<>	**Axis IV**
	Type: Acute, Chronic				
	Onset: Regular, Delayed				
ASD	**Acute Stress Disorder**	<>	<>	<>	
ANO	**Anorexia**	<>	<>	<>	**Axis V**
BUL	**Bulimia**	<>	<>	<>	current:
DEP	**Major Depressive Disorder**	<>	<>	<>	past year:
DYS	**Dysthymic Disorder**	<>	<>	<>	
MAN	**Mania**	<>	<>	<>	
HYPOMAN	**Hypomania**	<>	<>	<>	
ENU	**Enuresis**	<>	<>	<>	
	Type: Nocturnal, Diurnal, Both				
ENC	**Encopresis**	<>	<>	<>	
SCZ	**Schizophrenia**	<>	<>	<>	
PSY	**Psychosis**	<>	<>	<>	

Psychosocial Stressors:

Other Stressors:

Behavioral Observations

Appearance: Affect:

Effort: Level of Activity:

Unusual Behaviors:

Presenting Problem

Home

1.

2.

School

1.

2.

3.

4.

5.

Peers/Work

1.

2.

3.

4.

5.

Medication

Type:

Dosage:

ChIPS Scoring Form

Child's Name: _____

Date: _____

ADHD	ODD	CD

A. Inattention
  1. \<a> \<b>
  2. \< >
  3. \<a> \<b>
  4. \<a> \<b> \<c>
  5. \< >
  6. \< >
  7. \< >
  8. \<a> \<b>
  9. \<a> \<b>
 	
B. Hyperactivity–Impulsivity
  1. \<a> \<b>
  2. \<a> \<b>
  3. \< >
  4. \<a> \<b>
  5. \< >
  6. \<a> \<b>
  7. \< >
  8. \<a> \<b>
  9. \<a> \<b> \<c>
	1. \<a> \<b>
	2. \<a> \<b>
	3. \<a> \<b> \<c> \<d>
	4. \< >
	5. \<a> \<b>
	6. \< >
	7. \< >
	8. \< >
		1. \< >
		2. \<a> \<b>
		3. \< >
		4. \< >
		5. \< >
		6. \< >
		7. \<a> \<b>
		8. \<a> \<b>
		9. \< >
		10. \<a> \<b>
		11. \< >
		12. \< >
		13. \< >
		14. \< >
		15. \<a> \<b>

Criteria If ≥6 in *A only*, then criteria met Inattentive \< > If ≥6 in *B only*, then criteria met Hyperactive–Impulsive \< > If ≥6 in A *and* ≥6 in B, then criteria met Combined \< >	**Criteria** If ≥4, then criteria met ODD \< >	**Criteria** If ≥3, then criteria met CD \< >

Duration
1. _____ (years old)
2. \< > _____ (years old)
3. \< > _____ (months)
 	
  * DUR met for ADHD \< >
	Duration
	1. _____ (years old)
	2. \< > _____ (years old)
	3. \< > _____ (months)
	
	  * DUR met for ODD \< >
		Duration
		1. _____ (years old)
		2. \< > _____ (years old)
		3. \< > _____ (months)
		
		  * DUR met for CD \< >

Impairment 1. \< > home 2. \< > school 3. \< > peers	**Impairment** 1. \< > home 2. \< > school 3. \< > peers	**Impairment** 1. \< > home 2. \< > school 3. \< > peers
		Type Childhood Onset \< > Adolescent Onset \< > Mild \< > Moderate \< > Severe \< >

SUB AB	PHO	SOCIAL PHO

1. < >
    <a>_____
    <b>_____
    <c>_____
 	
    _____
2. < > _____
3. < > _____
4. < > _____
	1. _____
	    _____
	    _____
	2. <a> <b>
	3. <a> <b>
	4. <ai> <aii> <aiii> <aiv> <b>
	5. <a> <b>
		1. <a> <b>
		2. < >
		3. <a> <b>
		4. <ai> <aii> <aiii> <aiv> <b>
		5. < >

Duration
1. _____ (years old)
2. < > _____ (years old)
    _____ (months)
 	
  * DUR met for SUB AB < >
	Criteria
	    If 1–4, then criteria met
	           PHO < >
		Criteria
		    If 1–4, then criteria met
		       SOCIAL PHO < >

	Duration
	1. _____ (years old)
	2. < > _____ (years old)
	3. < > _____ (months)
	
	    * DUR met for PHO < >
		Duration
		1. _____ (years old)
		2. < > _____ (years old)
		3. < > _____ (months)
		
		  *DUR met for SOCIAL PHO < >

Impairment 1. <a> <b> 2. < > 3. <a> <b> 4. < >	**Impairment** 1. < > home 2. < > school 3. < > peers	**Impairment** 1. < > home 2. < > school 3. < > peers

Criteria
    If any use (Q1–4) and any
   impairment (1–4), then criteria
        met SUB AB < >
 	
Type(s) _____
_____
_____
_____
	Type(s)
	Animal < >
	Natural Environment < >
	Blood–Injection–Injury < >
	Situational < >
	Other _____ < >	

SEP ANX	GEN ANX	OCD

1. <a> <b>
2. <a> <b>
3. < >
4. <a> <b>
5. <a> <b>
6. <a> <b>
7. <a> <b>
8. <a> <b>
	1. < > _____
	 _____
	 _____
	 _____
	 _____
	2. <a> <b>
	3. <a> <b> <c> <d> <e> <f>
		A. Compulsions
		   1. < > _____
		   2. <a> _____
		      <b>
		   3. < >
		
		B. Obsessions
		   1. <a> _____
		      <b> _____
		      <c> _____
		   2. <a> <b> <c>
		   3. < >
		
		C. Interference
		   1. <a> <b> <c>

Criteria
   If ≥3, then criteria met
   SEP ANX < >
	Criteria
	   If 1–3, then criteria met
	   GEN ANX < >
		Criteria
		   If A1, A2, & C,
		   then criteria met
		   Compulsions < >
		
		   If B1, B2, & C,
		   then criteria met
		   Obsessions < >
		
		   If Compulsions +
		   and/or Obsessions +,
		   then criteria met
		   OCD < >

Duration
1. _____ (years old)
2. < > _____ (years old)
3. < > _____ (weeks)
 	
   *DUR met for SEP ANX < >
	Duration
	1. _____ (years old)
	2. < > _____ (years old)
	3. < > _____ (months)
	
	   *DUR met for GEN ANX < >
		Duration
		1. _____ (years old)
		2. < > _____ (years old)
		   _____ (months)
		
		   *DUR met for OCD < >

Impairment 1. < > home 2. < > school 3. < > peers	**Impairment** 1. < > home 2. < > school 3. < > peers	**Impairment** 1. < > home 2. < > school 3. < > peers

STRESS (ASD/PTSD)	ANO	BUL

A. Exposure
  1. <a> <b> _____
  2. <a> <b> <c> <d> <e>
  3. < > _____
B. Dissociation
  1. <a> <b> <c> <d>
  2. < >
  3. < >
  4. < >
  5. < >
C. Reexperiencing
  1. <a> <b> <c>
  2. <a> <b>
  3. <a> <b>
  4. <a> <b>
  5. < >
D. Avoidance
  1. <a> <b>
  2. <a> <b> <c>
  3. < >
  4. <a> <b>
  5. <a> <b>
  6. <a> <b>
  7. <a> <b>
E. Hyperarousal
  1. <a> <b>
  2. <a> <b>
  3. < >
  4. < >
  5. < >
	1. <a> <b>
	2. <a>
	   ht: _____
	   wt: _____
	  <b>
	   ht: _____
	   wt: _____
	3. <a> <b> <c>
	4. <a> <b> <c>
	5. < >
		1. < > _____
		_____
		2. <a> <b> <c> <d>
		3. <a> <b> <c> <d>
		4. <a> <b>

Criteria If A1 & A2, ≥3 in B, ≥1 in C, ≥3 in D, and ≥2 in E, then criteria met ASD < > If A1 & A2, ≥1 in C, ≥3 in D, and ≥2 in E, then criteria met PTSD < >	**Criteria** If 1–4 (&5 for pubescent girls), then criteria met ANO < >	**Criteria** If 1–4, then criteria met BUL < >

Duration
1. _____ (years old)
2. < > _____ (years old)
3. a. < > _____ (weeks)
   b. < >
   c. < > _____ (days)
4. < > _____ (months)
   *DUR met for ASD < >
   *DUR met for PTSD < >
	Duration
	1. _____ (years old)
	2. < > _____ (years old)
	3. < > _____ (months)
	
	   *DUR met for ANO < >
		Duration
		1. _____ (years old)
		2. < > _____ (years old)
		3. a. < > _____ (#/week)
		   b. < > _____ (months)
		
		   *DUR met for BUL < >

Impairment 1. < > home 2. < > school 3. < > peers	**Impairment** 1. < > home 2. < > school 3. < > peers	**Impairment** 1. < > home 2. < > school 3. < > peers
Type (PTSD) Acute < > Regular Onset < > Chronic < > Delayed Onset < >		

DEP/DYS (MDD/DD)	DEP/DYS (MDD/DD)	MAN/HYPOMAN

A. Dysphoric Mood
1. \<a\> \<b\> \<c\>
2. \<a\> \<bi\> \<bii\> \<biii\>
   \<c\> \<d\>
 	
B. Loss of Interest
1. \<a\> \<b\>
2. \<a\> \<b\> \<c\>
 	
C. Appetite Changes
1. \<a\> \<b\> \<c\>
2. \<a\> \<b\>
 	
D. Sleep Changes
   Bedtime: _____
   Wakeup: _____
1. \<a\> \<b\> \<c\>
2. \<a\> \<b\>
 	
E. Psychomotor Changes
1. \<a\> \<b\> \<c\> \<d\>
2. \<a\> \<b\>
 	
F. Low Energy
1. \<a\> \<b\> \<c\> \<d\>
 	
G. Guilt
1. \<a\> \<b\> \<c\> \<d\>
2. \<a\> \<b\>
 	
H. Impaired Concentration
1. \<a\> \<b\> \<c\> \<d\> \<e\>
2. \< \>
 	
I. Hopelessness
1. \<a\> \<b\> \<c\>
 	
J. Morbid/Suicidal Thoughts
1. \<a\> \<b\>
2. \<a\> \<b\> \<c\> \<d\> \<e\>
 	
_____
_____
_____
_____
_____
		A. Elevated Mood
		1. \<a\> _____
		   \<b\> _____
		   \<c\> _____
		2. \< \> _____
		
		B. Other Symptoms
		1. \<a\> _____
		   \<b\>
		2. \<a\> \<b\> \<c\> _____
		3. \<a\> \<b\> \<c\> \<d\>
		4. \<a\> \<b\> \<c\>
		5. \< \>
		6. \<a\> \<b\> \<c\> \<d\> \<e\>
		7. \<a\> \<b\> \<c\> \<d\>
		
		C. Interference
		1. \< \>
		2. \< \>

	Criteria If A &/or B & ≥5 of A–H or J, then criteria met MDD \< \> If A & ≥2 of C, D, F, G, H, or I, then criteria met DD \< \>	**Criteria** If A1(a, b, & c) + ≥3 in B + ≥1 in C *or* A2 + ≥4 in B + ≥1 in C, then criteria met MAN \< \> If A1(a, b, & c) + ≥3 in B + none in C *or* A2 + ≥4 in B + none in C, then criteria met HYPOMAN \< \>

	Duration
	1. _____ (years old)
	2. \< \> _____ (years old)
	3. MDD \< \> _____ (weeks)
	   DD \< \> _____ (months)
	
	*DUR met for MDD \< \>
	*DUR met for DD \< \>
		Duration
		1. _____ (years old)
		2. \< \> _____ (years old)
		3. MAN \< \> _____ (weeks)
		   HYPO \< \> _____ (days)
		
		*DUR met for MAN \< \>
		*DUR met for HYPOMAN \< \>

	Impairment 1. \< \> home 2. \< \> school 3. \< \> peers	**Impairment** 1. \< \> home 2. \< \> school 3. \< \> peers

ENU	SCZ/PSY	STRESSORS

ENU
 	
1. < >
2. <a> <b>
3. <a> <b>
 	
Criteria
   If 1, ≥1 in 2, 3a, and 3b,
   then criteria met
   ENU < >
 	
Duration
1. _____ (years old)
2. < > _____ (years old)
3. <a> _____ (x/week)
   <b> _____ (months)
 	
   *DUR met for ENU < >
 	
Impairment
1. < > home
2. < > school
3. < > peers
 	
Type
Nocturnal   < >
Diurnal   < >
Both   < >
	A. Psychotic Symptoms
	   1. <a> <b> <c> <d> <e>
	   2. <a> <b> <c> <d> <e> <f>
	   3. < >
	   4. < >
	   5. < >
	
	B. Interference
	   1. < >
	   2. < >
	   3. < >
	
	Criteria
	   If ≥2 in A and ≥1 in B,
	   then criteria met
	   SCZ < >
	
	   If ≥1 in A, then criteria met
	   PSY < >
	
	Duration
	1. _____ (years old)
	2. < > _____ (years old)
	3. < > _____ (months)
	
	   *DUR met for SCZ < >
	   *DUR met for PSY < >
		A. Child Abuse/Neglect
		1. <a> <b> <c>
		2. <a> <b> <c> <d>
		3. <a> <b> <c> <d>
		4. < >
		5. < >
		
		Duration
		1. _____
		2. < > _____
		3. _____
		4. _____
		5. < >
		
		B. Other Stressors
		   1. <a> <b> <c> <d> <e>
		   2. < >
		   3. <a> <b>
		   4. <a> <b> <c>
		   5. <a> <b>
		   6. <a> <b>
		   7. <a> _____
		        <b>
		   8. <a> <b> <c> <d>
		   9. < > _____
		        _____
		  10. < >
		  11. < > _____
		        _____
		        _____

ENC
 	
1. < >
2. < >
 	
Criteria
If both 1 & 2, then criteria met
   ENC < >
 	
Duration
1. _____ (years old)
2. < > _____ (years old)
3. <a> _____ (x/month)
   <b> _____ (months)
 	
   *DUR met for ENC < >
 	
Impairment
1. < > home
2. < > school
3. < > peers
	Impairment
	1. < > home
	2. < > school
	3. < > peers	

Child's Number: _____ Date: _____

Child's Name: _____ Time Started: _____

Date of Birth: _____ Age: _____ Time Ended: _____

Race: _____ Sex: _____ Interviewer: _____

Setting (circle one):   Inpatient,   Outpatient,   School,   Other Research Setting: _____

	Disorder	Symptoms	Diagnosis	Duration	Clinician's Diagnosis
ADHD	**Attention-Deficit/Hyperactivity Disorder** *Type:* Inattentive, Hyperactive–Impulsive, Combined	<>	<>	<>	Axis I
ODD	**Oppositional Defiant Disorder**	<>	<>	<>	
CD	**Conduct Disorder** *Onset:* Childhood, Adolescent *Severity:* Mild, Moderate, Severe	<>	<>	<>	
SUBAB	**Substance Abuse** *Substance(s):* _____	<>	<>	<>	
PHO	**Specific Phobia** *Type:* _____	<>	<>	<>	Axis II
SOCPHO	**Social Phobia**	<>	<>	<>	
SEPANX	**Separation Anxiety Disorder**	<>	<>	<>	Axis III
GENANX	**General Anxiety Disorder**	<>	<>	<>	
OCD	**Obsessive-Compulsive Disorder**	<>	<>	<>	
PTSD	**Posttraumatic Stress Disorder** *Type:* Acute, Chronic *Onset:* Regular, Delayed	<>	<>	<>	Axis IV
ASD	**Acute Stress Disorder**	<>	<>	<>	
ANO	**Anorexia**	<>	<>	<>	Axis V
BUL	**Bulimia**	<>	<>	<>	current:
DEP	**Major Depressive Disorder**	<>	<>	<>	past year:
DYS	**Dysthymic Disorder**	<>	<>	<>	
MAN	**Mania**	<>	<>	<>	
HYPOMAN	**Hypomania**	<>	<>	<>	
ENU	**Enuresis** *Type:* Nocturnal, Diurnal, Both	<>	<>	<>	
ENC	**Encopresis**	<>	<>	<>	
SCZ	**Schizophrenia**	<>	<>	<>	
PSY	**Psychosis**	<>	<>	<>	

Psychosocial Stressors:

Other Stressors:

Behavioral Observations

Appearance: Affect:

Effort: Level of Activity:

Unusual Behaviors:

Presenting Problem

Home

1.

2.

School

1.

2.

3.

4.

5.

Peers/Work

1.

2.

3.

4.

5.

Medication

Type:

Dosage:

ChIPS Scoring Form

ADHD	ODD	CD

A. Inattention
  1. \<a> \<b>
  2. \< >
  3. \<a> \<b>
  4. \<a> \<b> \<c>
  5. \< >
  6. \< >
  7. \< >
  8. \<a> \<b>
  9. \<a> \<b>
 	
B. Hyperactivity–Impulsivity
  1. \<a> \<b>
  2. \<a> \<b>
  3. \< >
  4. \<a> \<b>
  5. \< >
  6. \<a> \<b>
  7. \< >
  8. \<a> \<b>
  9. \<a> \<b> \<c>
	1. \<a> \<b>
	2. \<a> \<b>
	3. \<a> \<b> \<c> \<d>
	4. \< >
	5. \<a> \<b>
	6. \< >
	7. \< >
	8. \< >
		1. \< >
		2. \<a> \<b>
		3. \< >
		4. \< >
		5. \< >
		6. \< >
		7. \<a> \<b>
		8. \<a> \<b>
		9. \< >
		10. \<a> \<b>
		11. \< >
		12. \< >
		13. \< >
		14. \< >
		15. \<a> \<b>

Criteria If ≥6 in *A only*, then criteria met Inattentive \< > If ≥6 in *B only*, then criteria met Hyperactive–Impulsive \< > If ≥6 in A *and* ≥6 in B, then criteria met Combined \< >	**Criteria** If ≥4, then criteria met ODD \< >	**Criteria** If ≥3, then criteria met CD \< >

Duration
1. _____ (years old)
2. \< > _____ (years old)
3. \< > _____ (months)
 	
  * DUR met for ADHD \< >
	Duration
	1. _____ (years old)
	2. \< > _____ (years old)
	3. \< > _____ (months)
	
	  * DUR met for ODD \< >
		Duration
		1. _____ (years old)
		2. \< > _____ (years old)
		3. \< > _____ (months)
		
		  * DUR met for CD \< >

Impairment 1. \< > home 2. \< > school 3. \< > peers	**Impairment** 1. \< > home 2. \< > school 3. \< > peers	**Impairment** 1. \< > home 2. \< > school 3. \< > peers
		Type Childhood Onset \< > Adolescent Onset \< > Mild \< > Moderate \< > Severe \< >

SUB AB	PHO	SOCIAL PHO

1. < >
    <a>_____
    <b>_____
    <c>_____
 	
    _____
2. < > _____
3. < > _____
4. < > _____
	1. _____
	    _____
	    _____
	2. <a> <b>
	3. <a> <b>
	4. <ai> <aii> <aiii> <aiv> <b>
	5. <a> <b>
		1. <a> <b>
		2. < >
		3. <a> <b>
		4. <ai> <aii> <aiii> <aiv> <b>
		5. < >

Duration
1. _____ (years old)
2. < > _____ (years old)
    _____ (months)
 	
  * DUR met for SUB AB < >
	Criteria
	  If 1–4, then criteria met
	    PHO < >
		Criteria
		  If 1–4, then criteria met
		    SOCIAL PHO < >

	Duration
	1. _____ (years old)
	2. < > _____ (years old)
	3. < > _____ (months)
	
	  * DUR met for PHO < >
		Duration
		1. _____ (years old)
		2. < > _____ (years old)
		3. < > _____ (months)
		
		  *DUR met for SOCIAL PHO < >

Impairment 1. <a> <b> 2. < > 3. <a> <b> 4. < >	**Impairment** 1. < > home 2. < > school 3. < > peers	**Impairment** 1. < > home 2. < > school 3. < > peers

Criteria
  If any use (Q1–4) and any
  impairment (1–4), then criteria
    met SUB AB < >
 	
Type(s) _____
_____
_____
_____
	Type(s)
	Animal < >
	Natural Environment < >
	Blood–Injection–Injury < >
	Situational < >
	Other _____ < >	

SEP ANX	GEN ANX	OCD

1. \<a\> \<b\>
2. \<a\> \<b\>
3. \< \>
4. \<a\> \<b\>
5. \<a\> \<b\>
6. \<a\> \<b\>
7. \<a\> \<b\>
8. \<a\> \<b\>
	1. \< \> _____
	_____
	_____
	_____
	_____
	2. \<a\> \<b\>
	3. \<a\> \<b\> \<c\> \<d\> \<e\> \<f\>
		A. Compulsions
		   1. \< \> _____
		   2. \<a\> _____
		      \<b\>
		   3. \< \>
		
		B. Obsessions
		   1. \<a\> _____
		      \<b\> _____
		      \<c\> _____
		   2. \<a\> \<b\> \<c\>
		   3. \< \>
		
		C. Interference
		   1. \<a\> \<b\> \<c\>

Criteria
   If ≥3, then criteria met
     SEP ANX \< \>
	Criteria
	   If 1–3, then criteria met
	     GEN ANX \< \>
		Criteria
		   If A1, A2, & C,
		   then criteria met
		   Compulsions \< \>
		
		   If B1, B2, & C,
		   then criteria met
		   Obsessions \< \>
		
		   If Compulsions +
		   and/or Obsessions +,
		   then criteria met
		   OCD \< \>

Duration
1. _____ (years old)
2. \< \> _____ (years old)
3. \< \> _____ (weeks)
 	
  *DUR met for SEP ANX \< \>
	Duration
	1. _____ (years old)
	2. \< \> _____ (years old)
	3. \< \> _____ (months)
	
	  *DUR met for GEN ANX \< \>
		Duration
		1. _____ (years old)
		2. \< \> _____ (years old)
		   _____ (months)
		
		  *DUR met for OCD \< \>

Impairment 1. \< \> home 2. \< \> school 3. \< \> peers	**Impairment** 1. \< \> home 2. \< \> school 3. \< \> peers	**Impairment** 1. \< \> home 2. \< \> school 3. \< \> peers

STRESS (ASD/PTSD)	ANO	BUL

A. Exposure
  1. \<a> \<b> _____
  2. \<a> \<b> \<c> \<d> \<e>
  3. \< > _____
B. Dissociation
  1. \<a> \<b> \<c> \<d>
  2. \< >
  3. \< >
  4. \< >
  5. \< >
C. Reexperiencing
  1. \<a> \<b> \<c>
  2. \<a> \<b>
  3. \<a> \<b>
  4. \<a> \<b>
  5. \< >
D. Avoidance
  1. \<a> \<b>
  2. \<a> \<b> \<c>
  3. \< >
  4. \<a> \<b>
  5. \<a> \<b>
  6. \<a> \<b>
  7. \<a> \<b>
E. Hyperarousal
  1. \<a> \<b>
  2. \<a> \<b>
  3. \< >
  4. \< >
  5. \< >
	1. \<a> \<b>
	2. \<a>
	  ht: _____
	  wt: _____
	  \<b>
	  ht: _____
	  wt: _____
	3. \<a> \<b> \<c>
	4. \<a> \<b> \<c>
	5. \< >
		1. \< > _____
		_____
		2. \<a> \<b> \<c> \<d>
		3. \<a> \<b> \<c> \<d>
		4. \<a> \<b>

Criteria If A1 *&* A2, ≥3 in B, ≥1 in C, ≥3 in D, and ≥2 in E, then criteria met ASD \< > If A1 *&* A2, ≥1 in C, ≥3 in D, and ≥2 in E, then criteria met PTSD \< >	**Criteria** If 1–4 (&5 for pubescent girls), then criteria met ANO \< >	**Criteria** If 1–4, then criteria met BUL \< >

Duration
1. _____ (years old)
2. \< > _____ (years old)
3. a. \< > _____ (weeks)
   b. \< >
   c. \< > _____ (days)
4. \< > _____ (months)
   *DUR met for ASD \< >
   *DUR met for PTSD \< >
	Duration
	1. _____ (years old)
	2. \< > _____ (years old)
	3. \< > _____ (months)
	
	   *DUR met for ANO \< >
		Duration
		1. _____ (years old)
		2. \< > _____ (years old)
		3. a. \< > _____ (#/week)
		   b. \< > _____ (months)
		
		   *DUR met for BUL \< >

Impairment 1. \< > home 2. \< > school 3. \< > peers	**Impairment** 1. \< > home 2. \< > school 3. \< > peers	**Impairment** 1. \< > home 2. \< > school 3. \< > peers
Type (PTSD) Acute \< > Regular Onset \< > Chronic \< > Delayed Onset \< >		

DEP/DYS (MDD/DD)	DEP/DYS (MDD/DD)	MAN/HYPOMAN

A. Dysphoric Mood
  1. \<a> \<b> \<c>
  2. \<a> \<bi> \<bii> \<biii>
     \<c> \<d>
 	
B. Loss of Interest
  1. \<a> \<b>
  2. \<a> \<b> \<c>
 	
C. Appetite Changes
  1. \<a> \<b> \<c>
  2. \<a> \<b>
 	
D. Sleep Changes
     Bedtime: _____
     Wakeup: _____
  1. \<a> \<b> \<c>
  2. \<a> \<b>
 	
E. Psychomotor Changes
  1. \<a> \<b> \<c> \<d>
  2. \<a> \<b>
 	
F. Low Energy
  1. \<a> \<b> \<c> \<d>
 	
G. Guilt
  1. \<a> \<b> \<c> \<d>
  2. \<a> \<b>
 	
H. Impaired Concentration
  1. \<a> \<b> \<c> \<d> \<e>
  2. \< >
 	
I. Hopelessness
  1. \<a> \<b> \<c>
 	
J. Morbid/Suicidal Thoughts
  1. \<a> \<b>
  2. \<a> \<b> \<c> \<d> \<e>
 	
_____
_____
_____
_____
_____
		A. Elevated Mood
		  1. \<a> _____
		     \<b> _____
		     \<c> _____
		  2. \< > _____
		
		B. Other Symptoms
		  1. \<a> _____
		     \<b>
		  2. \<a> \<b> \<c> _____
		  3. \<a> \<b> \<c> \<d>
		  4. \<a> \<b> \<c>
		  5. \< >
		  6. \<a> \<b> \<c> \<d> \<e>
		  7. \<a> \<b> \<c> \<d>
		
		C. Interference
		  1. \< >
		  2. \< >

	Criteria If A &/or B & ≥5 of A–H or J, then criteria met MDD \< > If A & ≥2 of C, D, F, G, H, or I, then criteria met DD \< >	**Criteria** If A1(a, b, & c) + ≥3 in B + ≥1 in C *or* A2 + ≥4 in B + ≥1 in C, then criteria met MAN \< > If A1(a, b, & c) + ≥3 in B + none in C *or* A2 + ≥4 in B + none in C, then criteria met HYPOMAN \< >

	Duration
	1. _____ (years old)
	2. \< > _____ (years old)
	3. MDD \< > _____ (weeks)
	   DD \< > _____ (months)
	
	  *DUR met for MDD \< >
	  *DUR met for DD \< >
		Duration
		1. _____ (years old)
		2. \< > _____ (years old)
		3. MAN \< > _____ (weeks)
		   HYPO \< > _____ (days)
		
		  *DUR met for MAN \< >
		  *DUR met for HYPOMAN \< >

	Impairment 1. \< > home 2. \< > school 3. \< > peers	**Impairment** 1. \< > home 2. \< > school 3. \< > peers

ENU	SCZ/PSY	STRESSORS

1. < >
2. <a> <b>
3. <a> <b>
	A. Psychotic Symptoms
	  1. <a> <b> <c> <d> <e>
	  2. <a> <b> <c> <d> <e> <f>
	  3. < >
	  4. < >
	  5. < >
		A. Child Abuse/Neglect
		  1. <a> <b> <c>
		  2. <a> <b> <c> <d>
		  3. <a> <b> <c> <d>
		  4. < >
		  5. < >

Criteria
    If 1, ≥1 in 2, 3a, and 3b,
      then criteria met
        ENU < >
	B. Interference
	  1. < >
	  2. < >
	  3. < >
		Duration
		1. _____
		2. < > _____
		3. _____

Duration
1. _____ (years old)
2. < > _____ (years old)
3. <a> _____ (x/week)
   <b> _____ (months)
 	
   *DUR met for ENU < >
	Criteria
	    If ≥2 in A and ≥1 in B,
	      then criteria met
	        SCZ < >
	
	    If ≥1 in A, then criteria met
	        PSY < >
		4. _____
		5. < >

Impairment
1. < > home
2. < > school
3. < > peers
		B. Other Stressors
		  1. <a> <b> <c> <d> <e>
		  2. < >
		  3. <a> <b>
		  4. <a> <b> <c>
		  5. <a> <b>

Type
Nocturnal   < >
Diurnal   < >
Both   < >
	Duration
	1. _____ (years old)
	2. < > _____ (years old)
	3. < > _____ (months)
	
	   *DUR met for SCZ < >
	   *DUR met for PSY < >
		6. <a> <b>
		  7. <a> _____
		         <b>
		  8. <a> <b> <c> <d>
		  9. < > _____

ENC		
1. < > 2. < >	**Impairment** 1. < > home 2. < > school 3. < > peers	_____ _____ 10. < > 11. < > _____

Criteria
If both 1 & 2, then criteria met
        ENC < >
		_____
		      _____

Duration 1. _____ (years old) 2. < > _____ (years old) 3. <a> _____ (x/month) <b> _____ (months) *DUR met for ENC < >		
Impairment 1. < > home 2. < > school 3. < > peers		

ChIPS Scoring Form
Profile Sheet

Child's Number: _____   Date: _____

Child's Name: _____   Time Started: _____

Date of Birth: _____ Age: _____   Time Ended: _____

Race: _____ Sex: _____   Interviewer: _____

Setting (circle one):   Inpatient,   Outpatient,   School,   Other Research Setting: _____

	Disorder	Symptoms	Diagnosis	Duration	Clinician's Diagnosis
ADHD	**Attention-Deficit/Hyperactivity Disorder**	<>	<>	<>	Axis I
	Type: Inattentive, Hyperactive–Impulsive, Combined				
ODD	**Oppositional Defiant Disorder**	<>	<>	<>	
CD	**Conduct Disorder**	<>	<>	<>	
	Onset: Childhood, Adolescent				
	Severity: Mild, Moderate, Severe				
SUBAB	**Substance Abuse**	<>	<>	<>	
	Substance(s): _____				
PHO	**Specific Phobia**	<>	<>	<>	Axis II
	Type: _____				
SOCPHO	**Social Phobia**	<>	<>	<>	
SEPANX	**Separation Anxiety Disorder**	<>	<>	<>	Axis III
GENANX	**General Anxiety Disorder**	<>	<>	<>	
OCD	**Obsessive-Compulsive Disorder**	<>	<>	<>	
PTSD	**Posttraumatic Stress Disorder**	<>	<>	<>	Axis IV
	Type: Acute, Chronic				
	Onset: Regular, Delayed				
ASD	**Acute Stress Disorder**	<>	<>	<>	
ANO	**Anorexia**	<>	<>	<>	Axis V
BUL	**Bulimia**	<>	<>	<>	current:
DEP	**Major Depressive Disorder**	<>	<>	<>	past year:
DYS	**Dysthymic Disorder**	<>	<>	<>	
MAN	**Mania**	<>	<>	<>	
HYPOMAN	**Hypomania**	<>	<>	<>	
ENU	**Enuresis**	<>	<>	<>	
	Type: Nocturnal, Diurnal, Both				
ENC	**Encopresis**	<>	<>	<>	
SCZ	**Schizophrenia**	<>	<>	<>	
PSY	**Psychosis**	<>	<>	<>	

Psychosocial Stressors:

Other Stressors:

Behavioral Observations

Appearance: Affect:

Effort: Level of Activity:

Unusual Behaviors:

Presenting Problem

Home

1.

2.

School

1.

2.

3.

4.

5.

Peers/Work

1.

2.

3.

4.

5.

Medication

Type:

Dosage:

Child's Name: _____

Date: _____

ADHD	ODD	CD

A. Inattention
  1. \<a> \<b>
  2. \< >
  3. \<a> \<b>
  4. \<a> \<b> \<c>
  5. \< >
  6. \< >
  7. \< >
  8. \<a> \<b>
  9. \<a> \<b>
 	
B. Hyperactivity–Impulsivity
  1. \<a> \<b>
  2. \<a> \<b>
  3. \< >
  4. \<a> \<b>
  5. \< >
  6. \<a> \<b>
  7. \< >
  8. \<a> \<b>
  9. \<a> \<b> \<c>
	1. \<a> \<b>
	2. \<a> \<b>
	3. \<a> \<b> \<c> \<d>
	4. \< >
	5. \<a> \<b>
	6. \< >
	7. \< >
	8. \< >
		1. \< >
		2. \<a> \<b>
		3. \< >
		4. \< >
		5. \< >
		6. \< >
		7. \<a> \<b>
		8. \<a> \<b>
		9. \< >
		10. \<a> \<b>
		11. \< >
		12. \< >
		13. \< >
		14. \< >
		15. \<a> \<b>

Criteria If ≥6 in *A only*, then criteria met Inattentive \< > If ≥6 in *B only*, then criteria met Hyperactive–Impulsive \< > If ≥6 in A *and* ≥6 in B, then criteria met Combined \< >	**Criteria** If ≥4, then criteria met ODD \< >	**Criteria** If ≥3, then criteria met CD \< >

Duration
1. _____ (years old)
2. \< > _____ (years old)
3. \< > _____ (months)
 	
  * DUR met for ADHD \< >
	Duration
	1. _____ (years old)
	2. \< > _____ (years old)
	3. \< > _____ (months)
	
	  * DUR met for ODD \< >
		Duration
		1. _____ (years old)
		2. \< > _____ (years old)
		3. \< > _____ (months)
		
		  * DUR met for CD \< >

Impairment 1. \< > home 2. \< > school 3. \< > peers	**Impairment** 1. \< > home 2. \< > school 3. \< > peers	**Impairment** 1. \< > home 2. \< > school 3. \< > peers
		Type Childhood Onset \< > Adolescent Onset \< > Mild \< > Moderate \< > Severe \< >

SUB AB	PHO	SOCIAL PHO
1. < > 　　<a>_____ 　　<b>_____ 　　<c>_____ 　　_____ 2. < > _____ 3. < > _____ 4. < > _____	1. _____ 　　_____ 　　_____ 2. <a> <b> 3. <a> <b> 4. <ai> <aii> <aiii> <aiv> <b> 5. <a> <b>	1. <a> <b> 2. < > 3. <a> <b> 4. <ai> <aii> <aiii> <aiv> <b> 5. < >
Duration 1. _____ (years old) 2. < > _____ (years old) 　　_____ (months) 　　* DUR met for SUB AB < >	**Criteria** 　　If 1–4, then criteria met 　　　　PHO < >	**Criteria** 　　If 1–4, then criteria met 　　　SOCIAL PHO < >
(continued)	**Duration** 1. _____ (years old) 2. < > _____ (years old) 3. < > _____ (months) 　　* DUR met for PHO < >	**Duration** 1. _____ (years old) 2. < > _____ (years old) 3. < > _____ (months) 　*DUR met for SOCIAL PHO < >
Impairment 1. <a> <b> 2. < > 3. <a> <b> 4. < >	**Impairment** 1. < > home 2. < > school 3. < > peers	**Impairment** 1. < > home 2. < > school 3. < > peers
Criteria 　　If any use (Q1–4) and any 　impairment (1–4), then criteria 　　　　met SUB AB < > **Type(s)** _____ 　_____ 　_____ 　_____	**Type(s)** Animal　　　　　　　　　　 < > Natural Environment　　　 < > Blood–Injection–Injury　　 < > Situational　　　　　　　 < > Other _____　　 < >	

SEP ANX	GEN ANX	OCD

1. \<a\> \<b\>
2. \<a\> \<b\>
3. \< \>
4. \<a\> \<b\>
5. \<a\> \<b\>
6. \<a\> \<b\>
7. \<a\> \<b\>
8. \<a\> \<b\>
	1. \< \> _____
	    _____
	    _____
	    _____
	    _____
	
	2. \<a\> \<b\>
	3. \<a\> \<b\> \<c\> \<d\> \<e\> \<f\>
		A. Compulsions
		    1. \< \> _____
		    2. \<a\> _____
		       \<b\>
		    3. \< \>
		
		B. Obsessions
		    1. \<a\> _____
		       \<b\> _____
		       \<c\> _____
		    2. \<a\> \<b\> \<c\>
		    3. \< \>
		
		C. Interference
		    1. \<a\> \<b\> \<c\>

Criteria If ≥3, then criteria met SEP ANX \< \>	**Criteria** If 1–3, then criteria met GEN ANX \< \>	**Criteria** If A1, A2, & C, then criteria met Compulsions \< \> If B1, B2, & C, then criteria met Obsessions \< \> If Compulsions + and/or Obsessions +, then criteria met OCD \< \>
Duration 1. _____ (years old) 2. \< \> _____ (years old) 3. \< \> _____ (weeks) *DUR met for SEP ANX \< \>	**Duration** 1. _____ (years old) 2. \< \> _____ (years old) 3. \< \> _____ (months) *DUR met for GEN ANX \< \>	**Duration** 1. _____ (years old) 2. \< \> _____ (years old) _____ (months) *DUR met for OCD \< \>
Impairment 1. \< \> home 2. \< \> school 3. \< \> peers	**Impairment** 1. \< \> home 2. \< \> school 3. \< \> peers	**Impairment** 1. \< \> home 2. \< \> school 3. \< \> peers

STRESS (ASD/PTSD)	ANO	BUL

A. Exposure
  1. \<a> \<b> _____
  2. \<a> \<b> \<c> \<d> \<e>
  3. \< > _____
B. Dissociation
  1. \<a> \<b> \<c> \<d>
  2. \< >
  3. \< >
  4. \< >
  5. \< >
C. Reexperiencing
  1. \<a> \<b> \<c>
  2. \<a> \<b>
  3. \<a> \<b>
  4. \<a> \<b>
  5. \< >
D. Avoidance
  1. \<a> \<b>
  2. \<a> \<b> \<c>
  3. \< >
  4. \<a> \<b>
  5. \<a> \<b>
  6. \<a> \<b>
  7. \<a> \<b>
E. Hyperarousal
  1. \<a> \<b>
  2. \<a> \<b>
  3. \< >
  4. \< >
  5. \< >
	1. \<a> \<b>
	2. \<a>
	  ht: _____
	  wt: _____
	  \<b>
	  ht: _____
	  wt: _____
	3. \<a> \<b> \<c>
	4. \<a> \<b> \<c>
	5. \< >
		1. \< > _____
		_____
		2. \<a> \<b> \<c> \<d>
		3. \<a> \<b> \<c> \<d>
		4. \<a> \<b>

Criteria If A1 *&* A2, ≥3 in B, ≥1 in C, ≥3 in D, and ≥2 in E, then criteria met ASD \< > If A1 *&* A2, ≥1 in C, ≥3 in D, and ≥2 in E, then criteria met PTSD \< >	**Criteria** If 1–4 (&5 for pubescent girls), then criteria met ANO \< >	**Criteria** If 1–4, then criteria met BUL \< >

Duration
1. _____ (years old)
2. \< > _____ (years old)
3. a. \< > _____ (weeks)
  b. \< >
  c. \< > _____ (days)
4. \< > _____ (months)
    *DUR met for ASD \< >
    *DUR met for PTSD \< >
	Duration
	1. _____ (years old)
	2. \< > _____ (years old)
	3. \< > _____ (months)
	
	    *DUR met for ANO \< >
		Duration
		1. _____ (years old)
		2. \< > _____ (years old)
		3. a. \< > ____ (#/week)
		  b. \< > _____ (months)
		
		    *DUR met for BUL \< >

Impairment 1. \< > home 2. \< > school 3. \< > peers	**Impairment** 1. \< > home 2. \< > school 3. \< > peers	**Impairment** 1. \< > home 2. \< > school 3. \< > peers
Type (PTSD) Acute \< > Regular Onset \< > Chronic \< > Delayed Onset \< >		

DEP/DYS (MDD/DD)	DEP/DYS (MDD/DD)	MAN/HYPOMAN

A. Dysphoric Mood
  1. \<a> \<b> \<c>
  2. \<a> \<bi> \<bii> \<biii>
    \<c> \<d>
 	
B. Loss of Interest
  1. \<a> \<b>
  2. \<a> \<b> \<c>
 	
C. Appetite Changes
  1. \<a> \<b> \<c>
  2. \<a> \<b>
 	
D. Sleep Changes
    Bedtime: _____
    Wakeup: _____
  1. \<a> \<b> \<c>
  2. \<a> \<b>
 	
E. Psychomotor Changes
  1. \<a> \<b> \<c> \<d>
  2. \<a> \<b>
 	
F. Low Energy
  1. \<a> \<b> \<c> \<d>
 	
G. Guilt
  1. \<a> \<b> \<c> \<d>
  2. \<a> \<b>
 	
H. Impaired Concentration
  1. \<a> \<b> \<c> \<d> \<e>
  2. \< >
 	
I. Hopelessness
  1. \<a> \<b> \<c>
 	
J. Morbid/Suicidal Thoughts
  1. \<a> \<b>
  2. \<a> \<b> \<c> \<d> \<e>
 	
_____
_____
_____
_____
_____
		A. Elevated Mood
		  1. \<a> _____
		    \<b> _____
		    \<c> _____
		  2. \< > _____
		
		B. Other Symptoms
		  1. \<a> _____
		    \<b>
		  2. \<a> \<b> \<c> _____
		  3. \<a> \<b> \<c> \<d>
		  4. \<a> \<b> \<c>
		  5. \< >
		  6. \<a> \<b> \<c> \<d> \<e>
		  7. \<a> \<b> \<c> \<d>
		
		C. Interference
		  1. \< >
		  2. \< >

	Criteria If A &/or B & ≥5 of A–H or J, then criteria met MDD \< > If A & ≥2 of C, D, F, G, H, or I, then criteria met DD \< >	**Criteria** If A1(a, b, & c) + ≥3 in B + ≥1 in C *or* A2 + ≥4 in B + ≥1 in C, then criteria met MAN \< > If A1(a, b, & c) + ≥3 in B + none in C *or* A2 + ≥4 in B + none in C, then criteria met HYPOMAN \< >

	Duration
	1. _____ (years old)
	2. \< > _____ (years old)
	3. MDD \< > _____ (weeks)
	  DD \< > _____ (months)
	
	  *DUR met for MDD \< >
	  *DUR met for DD \< >
		Duration
		1. _____ (years old)
		2. \< > _____ (years old)
		3. MAN \< > _____ (weeks)
		  HYPO \< > _____ (days)
		
		  *DUR met for MAN \< >
		  *DUR met for HYPOMAN \< >

	Impairment 1. \< > home 2. \< > school 3. \< > peers	**Impairment** 1. \< > home 2. \< > school 3. \< > peers

ENU	SCZ/PSY	STRESSORS

1. < >
 2. <a> <b>
 3. <a> <b>
	A. Psychotic Symptoms
	   1. <a> <b> <c> <d> <e>
	   2. <a> <b> <c> <d> <e> <f>
	   3. < >
	   4. < >
	   5. < >
		A. Child Abuse/Neglect
		 1. <a> <b> <c>
		 2. <a> <b> <c> <d>
		 3. <a> <b> <c> <d>
		 4. < >
		 5. < >

ENU

1. < >
2. <a> <b>
3. <a> <b>

Criteria

    If 1, ≥1 in 2, 3a, and 3b,
        then criteria met
           ENU < >

Duration

1. _____ (years old)
2. < > _____ (years old)
3. <a> _____ (x/week)
   <b> _____ (months)

    *DUR met for ENU < >

Impairment

1. < > home
2. < > school
3. < > peers

Type

Nocturnal   < >
Diurnal   < >
Both   < >

ENC

1. < >
2. < >

Criteria

If both 1 & 2, then criteria met
          ENC < >

Duration

1. _____ (years old)
2. < > _____ (years old)
3. <a> _____ (x/month)
   <b> _____ (months)

    *DUR met for ENC < >

Impairment

1. < > home
2. < > school
3. < > peers

SCZ/PSY

A. Psychotic Symptoms
  1. <a> <b> <c> <d> <e>
  2. <a> <b> <c> <d> <e> <f>
  3. < >
  4. < >
  5. < >

B. Interference
  1. < >
  2. < >
  3. < >

Criteria

    If ≥2 in A and ≥1 in B,
      then criteria met
         SCZ < >

    If ≥1 in A, then criteria met
         PSY < >

Duration

1. _____ (years old)
2. < > _____ (years old)
3. < > _____ (months)

    *DUR met for SCZ < >
    *DUR met for PSY < >

Impairment

1. < > home
2. < > school
3. < > peers

STRESSORS

A. Child Abuse/Neglect
1. <a> <b> <c>
2. <a> <b> <c> <d>
3. <a> <b> <c> <d>
4. < >
5. < >

Duration

1. _____
2. < > _____
3. _____
4. _____
5. < >

B.   Other Stressors
  1.   <a> <b> <c> <d> <e>
  2.   < >
  3.   <a> <b>
  4.   <a> <b> <c>
  5.   <a> <b>
  6.   <a> <b>
  7.   <a> _____
       <b>
  8.   <a> <b> <c> <d>
  9.   < > _____

       _____

       _____

  10. < >
  11. < > _____

       _____

       _____

Child's Number: _____ Date: _____

Child's Name: _____ Time Started: _____

Date of Birth: _____ Age: _____ Time Ended: _____

Race: _____ Sex: _____ Interviewer: _____

Setting (circle one):   Inpatient,   Outpatient,   School,   Other Research Setting: _____

	Disorder	Symptoms	Diagnosis	Duration	Clinician's Diagnosis
ADHD	**Attention-Deficit/Hyperactivity Disorder**	<>	<>	<>	Axis I
	Type: Inattentive, Hyperactive–Impulsive, Combined				
ODD	**Oppositional Defiant Disorder**	<>	<>	<>	
CD	**Conduct Disorder**	<>	<>	<>	
	Onset: Childhood, Adolescent				
	Severity: Mild, Moderate, Severe				
SUBAB	**Substance Abuse**	<>	<>	<>	
	Substance(s): _____				
PHO	**Specific Phobia**	<>	<>	<>	Axis II
	Type: _____				
SOCPHO	**Social Phobia**	<>	<>	<>	
SEPANX	**Separation Anxiety Disorder**	<>	<>	<>	Axis III
GENANX	**General Anxiety Disorder**	<>	<>	<>	
OCD	**Obsessive-Compulsive Disorder**	<>	<>	<>	
PTSD	**Posttraumatic Stress Disorder**	<>	<>	<>	Axis IV
	Type: Acute, Chronic				
	Onset: Regular, Delayed				
ASD	**Acute Stress Disorder**	<>	<>	<>	
ANO	**Anorexia**	<>	<>	<>	Axis V
BUL	**Bulimia**	<>	<>	<>	current:
DEP	**Major Depressive Disorder**	<>	<>	<>	past year:
DYS	**Dysthymic Disorder**	<>	<>	<>	
MAN	**Mania**	<>	<>	<>	
HYPOMAN	**Hypomania**	<>	<>	<>	
ENU	**Enuresis**	<>	<>	<>	
	Type: Nocturnal, Diurnal, Both				
ENC	**Encopresis**	<>	<>	<>	
SCZ	**Schizophrenia**	<>	<>	<>	
PSY	**Psychosis**	<>	<>	<>	

Psychosocial Stressors:

Other Stressors:

Behavioral Observations

Appearance: Affect:

Effort: Level of Activity:

Unusual Behaviors:

Presenting Problem

Home

1.

2.

School

1.

2.

3.

4.

5.

Peers/Work

1.

2.

3.

4.

5.

Medication

Type:

Dosage:

ADHD	ODD	CD
A. Inattention 　1. <a> <b> 　2. < > 　3. <a> <b> 　4. <a> <b> <c> 　5. < > 　6. < > 　7. < > 　8. <a> <b> 　9. <a> <b> B. Hyperactivity–Impulsivity 　1. <a> <b> 　2. <a> <b> 　3. < > 　4. <a> <b> 　5. < > 　6. <a> <b> 　7. < > 　8. <a> <b> 　9. <a> <b> <c>	1. <a> <b> 2. <a> <b> 3. <a> <b> <c> <d> 4. < > 5. <a> <b> 6. < > 7. < > 8. < >	1.　< > 2.　<a> <b> 3.　< > 4.　< > 5.　< > 6.　< > 7.　<a> <b> 8.　<a> <b> 9.　< > 10.　<a> <b> 11.　< > 12.　< > 13.　< > 14.　< > 15.　<a> <b>
Criteria If ≥6 in *A only*, then criteria met Inattentive < > If ≥6 in *B only*, then criteria met Hyperactive–Impulsive < > If ≥6 in A *and* ≥6 in B, then criteria met Combined < >	**Criteria** If ≥4, then criteria met ODD < >	**Criteria** If ≥3, then criteria met CD < >
Duration 1. _____ (years old) 2. < > _____ (years old) 3. < > _____ (months) 　* DUR met for ADHD < >	**Duration** 1. _____ (years old) 2. < > _____ (years old) 3. < > _____ (months) 　* DUR met for ODD < >	**Duration** 1. _____ (years old) 2. < > _____ (years old) 3. < > _____ (months) 　* DUR met for CD < >
Impairment 1. < > home 2. < > school 3. < > peers	**Impairment** 1. < > home 2. < > school 3. < > peers	**Impairment** 1. < > home 2. < > school 3. < > peers
		Type Childhood Onset　< > Adolescent Onset　< > Mild　　　　　< > Moderate　　　< > Severe　　　　< >

SUB AB	PHO	SOCIAL PHO

1. < >
     \<a\>_____
     \<b\>_____
     \<c\>_____
 	
    _____
2. < > _____
3. < > _____
4. < > _____
	1. _____
	_____
	_____
	2. \<a\> \<b\>
	3. \<a\> \<b\>
	4. \<ai\> \<aii\> \<aiii\> \<aiv\> \<b\>
	5. \<a\> \<b\>
		1. \<a\> \<b\>
		2. < >
		3. \<a\> \<b\>
		4. \<ai\> \<aii\> \<aiii\> \<aiv\> \<b\>
		5. < >

Duration	Criteria	Criteria

1. _____ (years old)
2. < > _____ (years old)
    _____ (months)
 	
  * DUR met for SUB AB < >
	If 1–4, then criteria met
	          PHO < >
		If 1–4, then criteria met
		      SOCIAL PHO < >

	Duration	Duration
	1. _____ (years old) 2. < > _____ (years old) 3. < > _____ (months) * DUR met for PHO < >	1. _____ (years old) 2. < > _____ (years old) 3. < > _____ (months) *DUR met for SOCIAL PHO < >

Impairment	Impairment	Impairment
1. \<a\> \<b\> 2. < > 3. \<a\> \<b\> 4. < >	1. < > home 2. < > school 3. < > peers	1. < > home 2. < > school 3. < > peers

Criteria	Type(s)	
If any use (Q1–4) and any impairment (1–4), then criteria met SUB AB < > Type(s) _____ _____ _____ _____	Animal Natural Environment Blood–Injection–Injury Situational Other _____	< > < > < > < > < >

SEP ANX	GEN ANX	OCD

1. \<a\> \<b\>
2. \<a\> \<b\>
3. \< \>
4. \<a\> \<b\>
5. \<a\> \<b\>
6. \<a\> \<b\>
7. \<a\> \<b\>
8. \<a\> \<b\>
	1. \< \> _____
	_____
	_____
	_____
	_____
	2. \<a\> \<b\>
	3. \<a\> \<b\> \<c\> \<d\> \<e\> \<f\>
		A. Compulsions
		   1. \< \> _____
		   2. \<a\> _____
		      \<b\>
		   3. \< \>
		
		B. Obsessions
		   1. \<a\> _____
		      \<b\> _____
		      \<c\> _____
		   2. \<a\> \<b\> \<c\>
		   3. \< \>
		
		C. Interference
		   1. \<a\> \<b\> \<c\>

Criteria
 	
   If ≥3, then criteria met
     SEP ANX \< \>
	Criteria
	
	   If 1–3, then criteria met
	     GEN ANX \< \>
		Criteria
		   If A1, A2, & C,
		   then criteria met
		   Compulsions \< \>
		
		   If B1, B2, & C,
		   then criteria met
		   Obsessions \< \>
		
		   If Compulsions +
		   and/or Obsessions +,
		   then criteria met
		   OCD \< \>

Duration
1. _____ (years old)
2. \< \> _____ (years old)
3. \< \> _____ (weeks)
 	
  *DUR met for SEP ANX \< \>
	Duration
	1. _____ (years old)
	2. \< \> _____ (years old)
	3. \< \> _____ (months)
	
	  *DUR met for GEN ANX \< \>
		Duration
		1. _____ (years old)
		2. \< \> _____ (years old)
		     _____ (months)
		
		  *DUR met for OCD \< \>

Impairment 1. \< \> home 2. \< \> school 3. \< \> peers	**Impairment** 1. \< \> home 2. \< \> school 3. \< \> peers	**Impairment** 1. \< \> home 2. \< \> school 3. \< \> peers

STRESS (ASD/PTSD)	ANO	BUL

A. Exposure
  1. \<a\> \<b\> _____
  2. \<a\> \<b\> \<c\> \<d\> \<e\>
  3. \< \> _____
B. Dissociation
  1. \<a\> \<b\> \<c\> \<d\>
  2. \< \>
  3. \< \>
  4. \< \>
  5. \< \>
C. Reexperiencing
  1. \<a\> \<b\> \<c\>
  2. \<a\> \<b\>
  3. \<a\> \<b\>
  4. \<a\> \<b\>
  5. \< \>
D. Avoidance
  1. \<a\> \<b\>
  2. \<a\> \<b\> \<c\>
  3. \< \>
  4. \<a\> \<b\>
  5. \<a\> \<b\>
  6. \<a\> \<b\>
  7. \<a\> \<b\>
E. Hyperarousal
  1. \<a\> \<b\>
  2. \<a\> \<b\>
  3. \< \>
  4. \< \>
  5. \< \>
	1. \<a\> \<b\>
	2. \<a\>
	  ht: _____
	  wt: _____
	  \<b\>
	  ht: _____
	  wt: _____
	3. \<a\> \<b\> \<c\>
	4. \<a\> \<b\> \<c\>
	5. \< \>
		1. \< \> _____
		_____
		2. \<a\> \<b\> \<c\> \<d\>
		3. \<a\> \<b\> \<c\> \<d\>
		4. \<a\> \<b\>

Criteria If A1 & A2, ≥3 in B, ≥1 in C, ≥3 in D, and ≥2 in E, then criteria met ASD \< \> If A1 & A2, ≥1 in C, ≥3 in D, and ≥2 in E, then criteria met PTSD \< \>	**Criteria** If 1–4 (&5 for pubescent girls), then criteria met ANO \< \>	**Criteria** If 1–4, then criteria met BUL \< \>

Duration
1. _____ (years old)
2. \< \> _____ (years old)
3. a. \< \> _____ (weeks)
   b. \< \>
   c. \< \> _____ (days)
4. \< \> _____ (months)
    *DUR met for ASD \< \>
    *DUR met for PTSD \< \>
	Duration
	1. _____ (years old)
	2. \< \> _____ (years old)
	3. \< \> _____ (months)
	
	   *DUR met for ANO \< \>
		Duration
		1. _____ (years old)
		2. \< \> _____ (years old)
		3. a. \< \> ____ (#/week)
		   b. \< \> _____ (months)
		
		   *DUR met for BUL \< \>

Impairment 1. \< \> home 2. \< \> school 3. \< \> peers	**Impairment** 1. \< \> home 2. \< \> school 3. \< \> peers	**Impairment** 1. \< \> home 2. \< \> school 3. \< \> peers
Type (PTSD) Acute \< \> Regular Onset \< \> Chronic \< \> Delayed Onset \< \>		

DEP/DYS (MDD/DD)	DEP/DYS (MDD/DD)	MAN/HYPOMAN

A. Dysphoric Mood
  1. \<a> \<b> \<c>
  2. \<a> \<bi> \<bii> \<biii>
    \<c> \<d>
 	
B. Loss of Interest
  1. \<a> \<b>
  2. \<a> \<b> \<c>
 	
C. Appetite Changes
  1. \<a> \<b> \<c>
  2. \<a> \<b>
 	
D. Sleep Changes
    Bedtime: _____
    Wakeup: _____
  1. \<a> \<b> \<c>
  2. \<a> \<b>
 	
E. Psychomotor Changes
  1. \<a> \<b> \<c> \<d>
  2. \<a> \<b>
 	
F. Low Energy
  1. \<a> \<b> \<c> \<d>
 	
G. Guilt
  1. \<a> \<b> \<c> \<d>
  2. \<a> \<b>
 	
H. Impaired Concentration
  1. \<a> \<b> \<c> \<d> \<e>
  2. \< >
 	
I. Hopelessness
  1. \<a> \<b> \<c>
 	
J. Morbid/Suicidal Thoughts
  1. \<a> \<b>
  2. \<a> \<b> \<c> \<d> \<e>
 	
_____
_____
_____
_____
_____
		A. Elevated Mood
		  1. \<a> _____
		    \<b> _____
		    \<c> _____
		  2. \< > _____
		
		B. Other Symptoms
		  1. \<a> _____
		    \<b>
		  2. \<a> \<b> \<c> _____
		  3. \<a> \<b> \<c> \<d>
		  4. \<a> \<b> \<c>
		  5. \< >
		  6. \<a> \<b> \<c> \<d> \<e>
		  7. \<a> \<b> \<c> \<d>
		
		C. Interference
		  1. \< >
		  2. \< >

	Criteria If A &/or B & ≥5 of A–H or J, then criteria met MDD \< > If A & ≥2 of C, D, F, G, H, or I, then criteria met DD \< >	**Criteria** If A1(a, b, & c) + ≥3 in B + ≥1 in C *or* A2 + ≥4 in B + ≥1 in C, then criteria met MAN \< > If A1(a, b, & c) + ≥3 in B + none in C *or* A2 + ≥4 in B + none in C, then criteria met HYPOMAN \< >

	Duration
	1. _____ (years old)
	2. \< > _____ (years old)
	3. MDD \< > _____ (weeks)
	   DD \< > _____ (months)
	
	  *DUR met for MDD \< >
	  *DUR met for DD \< >
		Duration
		1. _____ (years old)
		2. \< > _____ (years old)
		3. MAN \< > _____ (weeks)
		   HYPO \< > _____ (days)
		
		  *DUR met for MAN \< >
		  *DUR met for HYPOMAN \< >

	Impairment 1. \< > home 2. \< > school 3. \< > peers	**Impairment** 1. \< > home 2. \< > school 3. \< > peers

ENU	SCZ/PSY	STRESSORS

1. < >
2. <a> <b>
3. <a> <b>
	A. Psychotic Symptoms
	  1. <a> <b> <c> <d> <e>
	  2. <a> <b> <c> <d> <e> <f>
	  3. < >
	  4. < >
	  5. < >
		A. Child Abuse/Neglect
		  1. <a> <b> <c>
		  2. <a> <b> <c> <d>
		  3. <a> <b> <c> <d>
		  4. < >
		  5. < >

Criteria
  If 1, ≥1 in 2, 3a, and 3b,
    then criteria met
      ENU < >

Duration
1. _____ (years old)
2. < > _____ (years old)
3. <a> _____ (x/week)
   <b> _____ (months)

  *DUR met for ENU < >

Impairment
1. < > home
2. < > school
3. < > peers

Type
Nocturnal   < >
Diurnal   < >
Both   < >

B. Interference
  1. < >
  2. < >
  3. < >

Criteria
  If ≥2 in A and ≥1 in B,
    then criteria met
      SCZ < >

  If ≥1 in A, then criteria met
      PSY < >

Duration
1. _____ (years old)
2. < > _____ (years old)
3. < > _____ (months)

  *DUR met for SCZ < >
  *DUR met for PSY < >

Impairment
1. < > home
2. < > school
3. < > peers

Duration
1. _____
2. < > _____
3. _____
4. _____
5. < >

B. Other Stressors
  1. <a> <b> <c> <d> <e>
  2. < >
  3. <a> <b>
  4. <a> <b> <c>
  5. <a> <b>
  6. <a> <b>
  7. <a> _____
      <b>
  8. <a> <b> <c> <d>
  9. < > _____
      _____
      _____
  10. < >
  11. < > _____
      _____
      _____

ENC

1. < >
2. < >

Criteria
If both 1 & 2, then criteria met
      ENC < >

Duration
1. _____ (years old)
2. < > _____ (years old)
3. <a> _____ (x/month)
   <b> _____ (months)

  *DUR met for ENC < >

Impairment
1. < > home
2. < > school
3. < > peers

ChIPS Scoring Form
Profile Sheet

Child's Number: _____ Date: _____

Child's Name: _____ Time Started: _____

Date of Birth: _____ Age: _____ Time Ended: _____

Race: _____ Sex: _____ Interviewer: _____

Setting (circle one):   Inpatient,   Outpatient,   School,   Other Research Setting: _____

	Disorder	Symptoms	Diagnosis	Duration	Clinician's Diagnosis
ADHD	**Attention-Deficit/Hyperactivity Disorder**	<>	<>	<>	Axis I
	Type: Inattentive, Hyperactive–Impulsive, Combined				
ODD	**Oppositional Defiant Disorder**	<>	<>	<>	
CD	**Conduct Disorder**	<>	<>	<>	
	Onset: Childhood, Adolescent				
	Severity: Mild, Moderate, Severe				
SUBAB	**Substance Abuse**	<>	<>	<>	
	Substance(s): _____				
PHO	**Specific Phobia**	<>	<>	<>	Axis II
	Type: _____				
SOCPHO	**Social Phobia**	<>	<>	<>	
SEPANX	**Separation Anxiety Disorder**	<>	<>	<>	Axis III
GENANX	**General Anxiety Disorder**	<>	<>	<>	
OCD	**Obsessive-Compulsive Disorder**	<>	<>	<>	
PTSD	**Posttraumatic Stress Disorder**	<>	<>	<>	Axis IV
	Type: Acute, Chronic				
	Onset: Regular, Delayed				
ASD	**Acute Stress Disorder**	<>	<>	<>	
ANO	**Anorexia**	<>	<>	<>	Axis V
BUL	**Bulimia**	<>	<>	<>	current:
DEP	**Major Depressive Disorder**	<>	<>	<>	past year:
DYS	**Dysthymic Disorder**	<>	<>	<>	
MAN	**Mania**	<>	<>	<>	
HYPOMAN	**Hypomania**	<>	<>	<>	
ENU	**Enuresis**	<>	<>	<>	
	Type: Nocturnal, Diurnal, Both				
ENC	**Encopresis**	<>	<>	<>	
SCZ	**Schizophrenia**	<>	<>	<>	
PSY	**Psychosis**	<>	<>	<>	

Psychosocial Stressors:

Other Stressors:

Behavioral Observations

Appearance: Affect:

Effort: Level of Activity:

Unusual Behaviors:

Presenting Problem

Home

1.

2.

School

1.

2.

3.

4.

5.

Peers/Work

1.

2.

3.

4.

5.

Medication

Type:

Dosage:

Child's Name: _____

Date: _____

ADHD	ODD	CD
A. Inattention	1. \<a> \<b>	1. \< >
1. \<a> \<b>	2. \<a> \<b>	2. \<a> \<b>
2. \< >	3. \<a> \<b> \<c> \<d>	3. \< >
3. \<a> \<b>	4. \< >	4. \< >
4. \<a> \<b> \<c>	5. \<a> \<b>	5. \< >
5. \< >	6. \< >	6. \< >
6. \< >	7. \< >	7. \<a> \<b>
7. \< >	8. \< >	8. \<a> \<b>
8. \<a> \<b>		9. \< >
9. \<a> \<b>		10. \<a> \<b>
		11. \< >
B. Hyperactivity–Impulsivity		12. \< >
1. \<a> \<b>		13. \< >
2. \<a> \<b>		14. \< >
3. \< >		15. \<a> \<b>
4. \<a> \<b>		
5. \< >		
6. \<a> \<b>		
7. \< >		
8. \<a> \<b>		
9. \<a> \<b> \<c>		

Criteria	**Criteria**	**Criteria**
If ≥6 in *A only*, then criteria met Inattentive \< > If ≥6 in *B only*, then criteria met Hyperactive–Impulsive \< > If ≥6 in A *and* ≥6 in B, then criteria met Combined \< >	If ≥4, then criteria met ODD \< >	If >3, then criteria met CD \< >

Duration	**Duration**	**Duration**
1. _____ (years old)	1. _____ (years old)	1. _____ (years old)
2. \< > _____ (years old)	2. \< > _____ (years old)	2. \< > _____ (years old)
3. \< > _____ (months)	3. \< > _____ (months)	3. \< > _____ (months)
* DUR met for ADHD \< >	* DUR met for ODD \< >	* DUR met for CD \< >

Impairment	**Impairment**	**Impairment**
1. \< > home	1. \< > home	1. \< > home
2. \< > school	2. \< > school	2. \< > school
3. \< > peers	3. \< > peers	3. \< > peers

Type
Childhood Onset \< >
Adolescent Onset \< >

Mild   \< >
Moderate   \< >
Severe   \< >

SUB AB	PHO	SOCIAL PHO

1. < >
     <a>_____
     <b>_____
     <c>_____
 	
     _____
 2. < > _____
 3. < > _____
 4. < > _____
	1. _____
	     _____
	     _____
	 2. <a> <b>
	 3. <a> <b>
	 4. <ai> <aii> <aiii> <aiv> <b>
	 5. <a> <b>
		1. <a> <b>
		 2. < >
		 3. <a> <b>
		 4. <ai> <aii> <aiii> <aiv> <b>
		 5. < >

SUB AB	PHO	SOCIAL PHO

Duration
 1. _____ (years old)
 2. < > _____ (years old)
     _____ (months)
 	
   * DUR met for SUB AB < >
	Criteria
	   If 1–4, then criteria met
	     PHO < >
		Criteria
		   If 1–4, then criteria met
		     SOCIAL PHO < >

	Duration
	 1. _____ (years old)
	 2. < > _____ (years old)
	 3. < > _____ (months)
	
	   * DUR met for PHO < >
		Duration
		 1. _____ (years old)
		 2. < > _____ (years old)
		 3. < > _____ (months)
		
		   *DUR met for SOCIAL PHO < >

SUB AB	PHO	SOCIAL PHO
Impairment 1. <a> <b> 2. < > 3. <a> <b> 4. < >	**Impairment** 1. < > home 2. < > school 3. < > peers	**Impairment** 1. < > home 2. < > school 3. < > peers

Criteria
   If any use (Q1–4) and any
 impairment (1–4), then criteria
     met SUB AB < >
 	
 Type(s) _____
 _____
 _____
 _____
	Type(s)
	 Animal < >
	 Natural Environment < >
	 Blood–Injection–Injury < >
	 Situational < >
	 Other _____ < >	

SEP ANX	GEN ANX	OCD

1. <a> <b>
 2. <a> <b>
 3. < >
 4. <a> <b>
 5. <a> <b>
 6. <a> <b>
 7. <a> <b>
 8. <a> <b>
	1. < > _____
	 _____
	 _____
	 _____
	 _____
	 2. <a> <b>
	 3. <a> <b> <c> <d> <e> <f>
		A. Compulsions
		   1. < > _____
		   2. <a> _____
		     <b>
		   3. < >
		
		 B. Obsessions
		   1. <a> _____
		     <b> _____
		     <c> _____
		   2. <a> <b> <c>
		   3. < >
		
		 C. Interference
		   1. <a> <b> <c>

Criteria If ≥3, then criteria met SEP ANX < >	**Criteria** If 1–3, then criteria met GEN ANX < >	**Criteria** If A1, A2, & C, then criteria met Compulsions < > If B1, B2, & C, then criteria met Obsessions < > If Compulsions + and/or Obsessions +, then criteria met OCD < >
Duration 1. _____ (years old) 2. < > _____ (years old) 3. < > _____ (weeks) *DUR met for SEP ANX < >	**Duration** 1. _____ (years old) 2. < > _____ (years old) 3. < > _____ (months) *DUR met for GEN ANX < >	**Duration** 1. _____ (years old) 2. < > _____ (years old) _____ (months) *DUR met for OCD < >
Impairment 1. < > home 2. < > school 3. < > peers	**Impairment** 1. < > home 2. < > school 3. < > peers	**Impairment** 1. < > home 2. < > school 3. < > peers

STRESS (ASD/PTSD)	ANO	BUL
A. Exposure 1. \<a> \<b> _____ 2. \<a> \<b> \<c> \<d> \<e> 3. \< > _____ B. Dissociation 1. \<a> \<b> \<c> \<d> 2. \< > 3. \< > 4. \< > 5. \< > C. Reexperiencing 1. \<a> \<b> \<c> 2. \<a> \<b> 3. \<a> \<b> 4. \<a> \<b> 5. \< > D. Avoidance 1. \<a> \<b> 2. \<a> \<b> \<c> 3. \< > 4. \<a> \<b> 5. \<a> \<b> 6. \<a> \<b> 7. \<a> \<b> E. Hyperarousal 1. \<a> \<b> 2. \<a> \<b> 3. \< > 4. \< > 5. \< >	1. \<a> \<b> 2. \<a> ht: _____ wt: _____ \<b> ht: _____ wt: _____ 3. \<a> \<b> \<c> 4. \<a> \<b> \<c> 5. \< >	1. \< > _____ _____ _ 2. \<a> \<b> \<c> \<d> 3. \<a> \<b> \<c> \<d> 4. \<a> \<b>
Criteria If A1 & A2, ≥3 in B, ≥1 in C, ≥3 in D, and ≥2 in E, then criteria met ASD \< > If A1 & A2, ≥1 in C, ≥3 in D, and ≥2 in E, then criteria met PTSD \< >	**Criteria** If 1–4 (&5 for pubescent girls), then criteria met ANO \< >	**Criteria** If 1–4, then criteria met BUL \< >
Duration 1. _____ (years old) 2. \< > _____ (years old) 3. a. \< > _____ (weeks) b. \< > c. \< > _____ (days) 4. \< > _____ (months) *DUR met for ASD \< > *DUR met for PTSD \< >	**Duration** 1. _____ (years old) 2. \< > _____ (years old) 3. \< > _____ (months) *DUR met for ANO \< >	**Duration** 1. _____ (years old) 2. \< > _____ (years old) 3. a. \< > _____ (#/week) b. \< > _____ (months) *DUR met for BUL \< >
Impairment 1. \< > home 2. \< > school 3. \< > peers	**Impairment** 1. \< > home 2. \< > school 3. \< > peers	**Impairment** 1. \< > home 2. \< > school 3. \< > peers
Type (PTSD) Acute \< > Regular Onset \< > Chronic \< > Delayed Onset \< >		

DEP/DYS (MDD/DD)	DEP/DYS (MDD/DD)	MAN/HYPOMAN

A. Dysphoric Mood
  1. \<a> \<b> \<c>
  2. \<a> \<bi> \<bii> \<biii>
    \<c> \<d>
 	
B. Loss of Interest
  1. \<a> \<b>
  2. \<a> \<b> \<c>
 	
C. Appetite Changes
  1. \<a> \<b> \<c>
  2. \<a> \<b>
 	
D. Sleep Changes
    Bedtime: _____
    Wakeup: _____
  1. \<a> \<b> \<c>
  2. \<a> \<b>
 	
E. Psychomotor Changes
  1. \<a> \<b> \<c> \<d>
  2. \<a> \<b>
 	
F. Low Energy
  1. \<a> \<b> \<c> \<d>
 	
G. Guilt
  1. \<a> \<b> \<c> \<d>
  2. \<a> \<b>
 	
H. Impaired Concentration
  1. \<a> \<b> \<c> \<d> \<e>
  2. \< >
 	
I. Hopelessness
  1. \<a> \<b> \<c>
 	
J. Morbid/Suicidal Thoughts
  1. \<a> \<b>
  2. \<a> \<b> \<c> \<d> \<e>
 	
_____
_____
_____
_____
_____
	Criteria
	If A &/or B & $\geq$5 of A–H or J,
	then criteria met
	MDD \< >
	
	If A & $\geq$2 of C, D, F, G, H, or I,
	then criteria met
	DD \< >
	
	--- 	
	
	Duration
	1. _____ (years old)
	2. \< > _____ (years old)
	3. MDD \< > _____ (weeks)
	   DD \< > _____ (months)
	
	  *DUR met for MDD \< >
	  *DUR met for DD \< >
	
	--- 	
	
	Impairment
	1. \< > home
	2. \< > school
	3. \< > peers
		A. Elevated Mood
		  1. \<a> _____
		    \<b> _____
		    \<c> _____
		  2. \< > _____
		
		B. Other Symptoms
		  1. \<a> _____
		    \<b>
		  2. \<a> \<b> \<c> _____
		  3. \<a> \<b> \<c> \<d>
		  4. \<a> \<b> \<c>
		  5. \< >
		  6. \<a> \<b> \<c> \<d> \<e>
		  7. \<a> \<b> \<c> \<d>
		
		C. Interference
		  1. \< >
		  2. \< >
		
		Criteria
		If A1(a, b, & c) + $\geq$3 in B + $\geq$1 in C
		or
		A2 + $\geq$4 in B + $\geq$1 in C,
		then criteria met
		MAN \< >
		
		If A1(a, b, & c) + $\geq$3 in B +
		none in C
		or
		A2 + $\geq$4 in B + none in C,
		then criteria met
		HYPOMAN \< >
		
		--- 	
		
		Duration
		1. _____ (years old)
		2. \< > _____ (years old)
		3. MAN \< > _____ (weeks)
		   HYPO \< > _____ (days)
		
		  *DUR met for MAN \< >
		  *DUR met for HYPOMAN \< >
		
		--- 	
		
		Impairment
		1. \< > home
		2. \< > school
		3. \< > peers

ENU	SCZ/PSY	STRESSORS

1. < >
 2. <a> <b>
 3. <a> <b>
	A. Psychotic Symptoms
	   1. <a> <b> <c> <d> <e>
	   2. <a> <b> <c> <d> <e> <f>
	   3. < >
	   4. < >
	   5. < >
		A. Child Abuse/Neglect
		   1. <a> <b> <c>
		   2. <a> <b> <c> <d>
		   3. <a> <b> <c> <d>
		   4. < >
		   5. < >

ENU

1. < >
2. <a> <b>
3. <a> <b>

Criteria

    If 1, ≥1 in 2, 3a, and 3b,
      then criteria met
          ENU < >

Duration

1. _____ (years old)
2. < > _____ (years old)
3. <a> _____ (x/week)
   <b> _____ (months)

    *DUR met for ENU < >

Impairment

1. < > home
2. < > school
3. < > peers

Type

Nocturnal   < >
Diurnal   < >
Both   < >

ENC

1. < >
2. < >

Criteria

If both 1 & 2, then criteria met
         ENC < >

Duration

1. _____ (years old)
2. < > _____ (years old)
3. <a> _____ (x/month)
   <b> _____ (months)

    *DUR met for ENC < >

Impairment

1. < > home
2. < > school
3. < > peers

SCZ/PSY

A. Psychotic Symptoms
  1. <a> <b> <c> <d> <e>
  2. <a> <b> <c> <d> <e> <f>
  3. < >
  4. < >
  5. < >

B. Interference
  1. < >
  2. < >
  3. < >

Criteria

    If ≥2 in A and ≥1 in B,
      then criteria met
         SCZ < >

    If ≥1 in A, then criteria met
         PSY < >

Duration

1. _____ (years old)
2. < > _____ (years old)
3. < > _____ (months)

    *DUR met for SCZ < >
    *DUR met for PSY < >

Impairment

1. < > home
2. < > school
3. < > peers

STRESSORS

A. Child Abuse/Neglect
  1. <a> <b> <c>
  2. <a> <b> <c> <d>
  3. <a> <b> <c> <d>
  4. < >
  5. < >

Duration

1. _____
2. < > _____
3. _____
4. _____
5. < >

B.   Other Stressors
  1.   <a> <b> <c> <d> <e>
  2.   < >
  3.   <a> <b>
  4.   <a> <b> <c>
  5.   <a> <b>
  6.   <a> <b>
  7.   <a> _____
       <b>
  8.   <a> <b> <c> <d>
  9.   < > _____
          _____
  10. < >
  11. < > _____
          _____
          _____

Child's Number: _____ Date: _____

Child's Name: _____ Time Started: _____

Date of Birth: _____ Age: _____ Time Ended: _____

Race: _____ Sex: _____ Interviewer: _____

Setting (circle one):   Inpatient,   Outpatient,   School,   Other Research Setting: _____

	Disorder	Symptoms	Diagnosis	Duration	Clinician's Diagnosis
ADHD	**Attention-Deficit/Hyperactivity Disorder**	<>	<>	<>	Axis I
	Type: Inattentive, Hyperactive–Impulsive, Combined				
ODD	**Oppositional Defiant Disorder**	<>	<>	<>	
CD	**Conduct Disorder**	<>	<>	<>	
	Onset: Childhood, Adolescent				
	Severity: Mild, Moderate, Severe				
SUBAB	**Substance Abuse**	<>	<>	<>	
	Substance(s): _____				
PHO	**Specific Phobia**	<>	<>	<>	Axis II
	Type: _____				
SOCPHO	**Social Phobia**	<>	<>	<>	
SEPANX	**Separation Anxiety Disorder**	<>	<>	<>	Axis III
GENANX	**General Anxiety Disorder**	<>	<>	<>	
OCD	**Obsessive-Compulsive Disorder**	<>	<>	<>	
PTSD	**Posttraumatic Stress Disorder**	<>	<>	<>	Axis IV
	Type: Acute, Chronic				
	Onset: Regular, Delayed				
ASD	**Acute Stress Disorder**	<>	<>	<>	
ANO	**Anorexia**	<>	<>	<>	Axis V
BUL	**Bulimia**	<>	<>	<>	current:
DEP	**Major Depressive Disorder**	<>	<>	<>	past year:
DYS	**Dysthymic Disorder**	<>	<>	<>	
MAN	**Mania**	<>	<>	<>	
HYPOMAN	**Hypomania**	<>	<>	<>	
ENU	**Enuresis**	<>	<>	<>	
	Type: Nocturnal, Diurnal, Both				
ENC	**Encopresis**	<>	<>	<>	
SCZ	**Schizophrenia**	<>	<>	<>	
PSY	**Psychosis**	<>	<>	<>	

Psychosocial Stressors:

Other Stressors:

Behavioral Observations

Appearance: Affect:

Effort: Level of Activity:

Unusual Behaviors:

Presenting Problem

Home

1.

2.

School

1.

2.

3.

4.

5.

Peers/Work

1.

2.

3.

4.

5.

Medication

Type:

Dosage:

ADHD	ODD	CD
A. Inattention 　1. \<a> \<b> 　2. \< > 　3. \<a> \<b> 　4. \<a> \<b> \<c> 　5. \< > 　6. \< > 　7. \< > 　8. \<a> \<b> 　9. \<a> \<b> B. Hyperactivity–Impulsivity 　1. \<a> \<b> 　2. \<a> \<b> 　3. \< > 　4. \<a> \<b> 　5. \< > 　6. \<a> \<b> 　7. \< > 　8. \<a> \<b> 　9. \<a> \<b> \<c>	1. \<a> \<b> 2. \<a> \<b> 3. \<a> \<b> \<c> \<d> 4. \< > 5. \<a> \<b> 6. \< > 7. \< > 8. \< >	1. \< > 2. \<a> \<b> 3. \< > 4. \< > 5. \< > 6. \< > 7. \<a> \<b> 8. \<a> \<b> 9. \< > 10. \<a> \<b> 11. \< > 12. \< > 13. \< > 14. \< > 15. \<a> \<b>
Criteria 　If ≥6 in *A only*, then criteria met 　　Inattentive \< > 　If ≥6 in *B only*, then criteria met 　　Hyperactive–Impulsive \< > 　　If ≥6 in A *and* ≥6 in B, 　　then criteria met 　　Combined \< >	**Criteria** 　If ≥4, then criteria met 　　ODD \< >	**Criteria** 　If ≥3, then criteria met 　　CD \< >
Duration 1. _____ (years old) 2. \< > _____ (years old) 3. \< > _____ (months) 　* DUR met for ADHD \< >	**Duration** 1. _____ (years old) 2. \< > _____ (years old) 3. \< > _____ (months) 　* DUR met for ODD \< >	**Duration** 1. _____ (years old) 2. \< > _____ (years old) 3. \< > _____ (months) 　* DUR met for CD \< >
Impairment 1. \< > home 2. \< > school 3. \< > peers	**Impairment** 1. \< > home 2. \< > school 3. \< > peers	**Impairment** 1. \< > home 2. \< > school 3. \< > peers
		Type Childhood Onset　\< > Adolescent Onset　\< > Mild　　　　　　\< > Moderate　　　　\< > Severe　　　　　\< >

SUB AB	PHO	SOCIAL PHO
1. < > 　　<a>_____ 　　<b>_____ 　　<c>_____ 　　_____ 2. < > _____ 3. < > _____ 4. < > _____	1. _____ 　　_____ 　　_____ 2. <a> <b> 3. <a> <b> 4. <ai> <aii> <aiii> <aiv> <b> 5. <a> <b>	1. <a> <b> 2. < > 3. <a> <b> 4. <ai> <aii> <aiii> <aiv> <b> 5. < >
Duration 1. _____ (years old) 2. < > _____ (years old) 　　_____ (months) 　* DUR met for SUB AB < >	**Criteria** 　If 1–4, then criteria met 　　　PHO < >	**Criteria** 　If 1–4, then criteria met 　　SOCIAL PHO < >
	Duration 1. _____ (years old) 2. < > _____ (years old) 3. < > _____ (months) 　* DUR met for PHO < >	**Duration** 1. _____ (years old) 2. < > _____ (years old) 3. < > _____ (months) 　*DUR met for SOCIAL PHO < >
Impairment 1. <a> <b> 2. < > 3. <a> <b> 4. < >	**Impairment** 1. < > home 2. < > school 3. < > peers	**Impairment** 1. < > home 2. < > school 3. < > peers
Criteria 　If any use (Q1–4) and any 　impairment (1–4), then criteria 　　met SUB AB < > **Type(s)** _____ _____ _____ _____	**Type(s)** Animal　　　　　　　　< > Natural Environment　< > Blood–Injection–Injury　< > Situational　　　　　　< > Other _____　< >	

SEP ANX	GEN ANX	OCD
1. <a> <b> 2. <a> <b> 3. < > 4. <a> <b> 5. <a> <b> 6. <a> <b> 7. <a> <b> 8. <a> <b>	1. < > _____ _____ _____ _____ _____ 2. <a> <b> 3. <a> <b> <c> <d> <e> <f>	A. Compulsions 1. < > _____ 2. <a> _____ <b> 3. < > B. Obsessions 1. <a> _____ <b> _____ <c> _____ 2. <a> <b> <c> 3. < > C. Interference 1. <a> <b> <c>
Criteria If ≥3, then criteria met SEP ANX < >	**Criteria** If 1–3, then criteria met GEN ANX < >	**Criteria** If A1, A2, & C, then criteria met Compulsions < > If B1, B2, & C, then criteria met Obsessions < > If Compulsions + and/or Obsessions +, then criteria met OCD < >
Duration 1. _____ (years old) 2. < > _____ (years old) 3. < > _____ (weeks) *DUR met for SEP ANX < >	**Duration** 1. _____ (years old) 2. < > _____ (years old) 3. < > _____ (months) *DUR met for GEN ANX < >	**Duration** 1. _____ (years old) 2. < > _____ (years old) _____ (months) *DUR met for OCD < >
Impairment 1. < > home 2. < > school 3. < > peers	**Impairment** 1. < > home 2. < > school 3. < > peers	**Impairment** 1. < > home 2. < > school 3. < > peers

STRESS (ASD/PTSD)	ANO	BUL

A. Exposure
    1. \<a> \<b> _____
    2. \<a> \<b> \<c> \<d> \<e>
    3. \< > _____
B. Dissociation
    1. \<a> \<b> \<c> \<d>
    2. \< >
    3. \< >
    4. \< >
    5. \< >
C. Reexperiencing
    1. \<a> \<b> \<c>
    2. \<a> \<b>
    3. \<a> \<b>
    4. \<a> \<b>
    5. \< >
D. Avoidance
    1. \<a> \<b>
    2. \<a> \<b> \<c>
    3. \< >
    4. \<a> \<b>
    5. \<a> \<b>
    6. \<a> \<b>
    7. \<a> \<b>
E. Hyperarousal
    1. \<a> \<b>
    2. \<a> \<b>
    3. \< >
    4. \< >
    5. \< >
	1. \<a> \<b>
	2. \<a>
	    ht: _____
	    wt: _____
	    \<b>
	    ht: _____
	    wt: _____
	3. \<a> \<b> \<c>
	4. \<a> \<b> \<c>
	5. \< >
		1. \< > _____
		_____
		_
		2. \<a> \<b> \<c> \<d>
		3. \<a> \<b> \<c> \<d>
		4. \<a> \<b>

Criteria If A1 & A2, ≥3 in B, ≥1 in C, ≥3 in D, and ≥2 in E, then criteria met ASD \< > If A1 & A2, ≥1 in C, ≥3 in D, and ≥2 in E, then criteria met PTSD \< >	**Criteria** If 1–4 (&5 for pubescent girls), then criteria met ANO \< >	**Criteria** If 1–4, then criteria met BUL \< >

Duration
1. _____ (years old)
2. \< > _____ (years old)
3. a. \< > _____ (weeks)
    b. \< >
    c. \< > _____ (days)
4. \< > _____ (months)
        *DUR met for ASD \< >
        *DUR met for PTSD \< >
	Duration
	1. _____ (years old)
	2. \< > _____ (years old)
	3. \< > _____ (months)
	
	    *DUR met for ANO \< >
		Duration
		1. _____ (years old)
		2. \< > _____ (years old)
		3. a. \< > _____ (#/week)
		    b. \< > _____ (months)
		
		    *DUR met for BUL \< >

Impairment 1. \< > home 2. \< > school 3. \< > peers	**Impairment** 1. \< > home 2. \< > school 3. \< > peers	**Impairment** 1. \< > home 2. \< > school 3. \< > peers
Type (PTSD) Acute \< > Regular Onset \< > Chronic \< > Delayed Onset \< >		

DEP/DYS (MDD/DD)	DEP/DYS (MDD/DD)	MAN/HYPOMAN

A. Dysphoric Mood
  1. \<a> \<b> \<c>
  2. \<a> \<bi> \<bii> \<biii>
     \<c> \<d>
 	
B. Loss of Interest
  1. \<a> \<b>
  2. \<a> \<b> \<c>
 	
C. Appetite Changes
  1. \<a> \<b> \<c>
  2. \<a> \<b>
 	
D. Sleep Changes
     Bedtime: _____
     Wakeup: _____
  1. \<a> \<b> \<c>
  2. \<a> \<b>
 	
E. Psychomotor Changes
  1. \<a> \<b> \<c> \<d>
  2. \<a> \<b>
 	
F. Low Energy
  1. \<a> \<b> \<c> \<d>
 	
G. Guilt
  1. \<a> \<b> \<c> \<d>
  2. \<a> \<b>
 	
H. Impaired Concentration
  1. \<a> \<b> \<c> \<d> \<e>
  2. \< >
 	
I. Hopelessness
  1. \<a> \<b> \<c>
 	
J. Morbid/Suicidal Thoughts
  1. \<a> \<b>
  2. \<a> \<b> \<c> \<d> \<e>
 	
_____
_____
_____
_____
_____
		A. Elevated Mood
		  1. \<a> _____
		     \<b> _____
		     \<c> _____
		  2. \< > _____
		
		B. Other Symptoms
		  1. \<a> _____
		     \<b>
		  2. \<a> \<b> \<c> _____
		  3. \<a> \<b> \<c> \<d>
		  4. \<a> \<b> \<c>
		  5. \< >
		  6. \<a> \<b> \<c> \<d> \<e>
		  7. \<a> \<b> \<c> \<d>
		
		C. Interference
		  1. \< >
		  2. \< >

	Criteria If A &/or B & ≥5 of A–H or J, then criteria met MDD \< > If A & ≥2 of C, D, F, G, H, or I, then criteria met DD \< >	**Criteria** If A1(a, b, & c) + ≥3 in B + ≥1 in C *or* A2 + ≥4 in B + ≥1 in C, then criteria met MAN \< > If A1(a, b, & c) + ≥3 in B + none in C *or* A2 + ≥4 in B + none in C, then criteria met HYPOMAN \< >

	Duration
	1. _____ (years old)
	2. \< > _____ (years old)
	3. MDD \< > _____ (weeks)
	    DD \< > _____ (months)
	
	   *DUR met for MDD \< >
	   *DUR met for DD \< >
		Duration
		1. _____ (years old)
		2. \< > _____ (years old)
		3. MAN \< > _____ (weeks)
		    HYPO \< > _____ (days)
		
		   *DUR met for MAN \< >
		   *DUR met for HYPOMAN \< >

	Impairment 1. \< > home 2. \< > school 3. \< > peers	**Impairment** 1. \< > home 2. \< > school 3. \< > peers

ENU	SCZ/PSY	STRESSORS
1. < > 2. <a> <b> 3. <a> <b>	A. Psychotic Symptoms 　1. <a> <b> <c> <d> <e> 　2. <a> <b> <c> <d> <e> <f> 　3. < > 　4. < > 　5. < >	A. Child Abuse/Neglect 　1. <a> <b> <c> 　2. <a> <b> <c> <d> 　3. <a> <b> <c> <d> 　4. < > 　5. < >
Criteria 　If 1, ≥1 in 2, 3a, and 3b, 　　then criteria met 　　　ENU < >	B. Interference 　1. < > 　2. < > 　3. < >	**Duration** 1. _____ 2. < > _____ 3. _____ 4. _____ 5. < >
Duration 1. _____ (years old) 2. < > _____ (years old) 3. <a> _____ (x/week) 　<b> _____ (months) 　*DUR met for ENU < >	**Criteria** 　If ≥2 in A and ≥1 in B, 　　then criteria met 　　　SCZ < > 　If ≥1 in A, then criteria met 　　　PSY < >	B.　Other Stressors 　1.　<a> <b> <c> <d> <e> 　2.　< > 　3.　<a> <b> 　4.　<a> <b> <c> 　5.　<a> <b> 　6.　<a> <b>
Impairment 1. < > home 2. < > school 3. < > peers		7.　<a> _____ 　　　<b> 　8.　<a> <b> <c> <d> 　9.　< > _____
Type Nocturnal　　　　< > Diurnal　　　　　< > Both　　　　　　< >	**Duration** 1. _____ (years old) 2. < > _____ (years old) 3. < > _____ (months) 　*DUR met for SCZ < > 　*DUR met for PSY < >	_____ _____ 　10.　< > 　11.　< > _____
ENC		_____
1. < > 2. < >	**Impairment** 1. < > home 2. < > school 3. < > peers	_____
Criteria If both 1 & 2, then criteria met 　　　ENC < >		
Duration 1. _____ (years old) 2. < > _____ (years old) 3. <a> _____ (x/month) 　<b> _____ (months) 　*DUR met for ENC < >		
Impairment 1. < > home 2. < > school 3. < > peers		

Child's Number: _____ Date: _____

Child's Name: _____ Time Started: _____

Date of Birth: _____ Age: _____ Time Ended: _____

Race: _____ Sex: _____ Interviewer: _____

Setting (circle one):   Inpatient,   Outpatient,   School,   Other Research Setting: _____

	Disorder	Symptoms	Diagnosis	Duration	Clinician's Diagnosis
ADHD	**Attention-Deficit/Hyperactivity Disorder**	<>	<>	<>	Axis I
	Type: Inattentive, Hyperactive–Impulsive, Combined				
ODD	**Oppositional Defiant Disorder**	<>	<>	<>	
CD	**Conduct Disorder**	<>	<>	<>	
	Onset: Childhood, Adolescent				
	Severity: Mild, Moderate, Severe				
SUBAB	**Substance Abuse**	<>	<>	<>	
	Substance(s): _____				
PHO	**Specific Phobia**	<>	<>	<>	Axis II
	Type: _____				
SOCPHO	**Social Phobia**	<>	<>	<>	
SEPANX	**Separation Anxiety Disorder**	<>	<>	<>	Axis III
GENANX	**General Anxiety Disorder**	<>	<>	<>	
OCD	**Obsessive-Compulsive Disorder**	<>	<>	<>	
PTSD	**Posttraumatic Stress Disorder**	<>	<>	<>	Axis IV
	Type: Acute, Chronic				
	Onset: Regular, Delayed				
ASD	**Acute Stress Disorder**	<>	<>	<>	
ANO	**Anorexia**	<>	<>	<>	Axis V
BUL	**Bulimia**	<>	<>	<>	current:
DEP	**Major Depressive Disorder**	<>	<>	<>	past year:
DYS	**Dysthymic Disorder**	<>	<>	<>	
MAN	**Mania**	<>	<>	<>	
HYPOMAN	**Hypomania**	<>	<>	<>	
ENU	**Enuresis**	<>	<>	<>	
	Type: Nocturnal, Diurnal, Both				
ENC	**Encopresis**	<>	<>	<>	
SCZ	**Schizophrenia**	<>	<>	<>	
PSY	**Psychosis**	<>	<>	<>	

Psychosocial Stressors:

Other Stressors:

Behavioral Observations

Appearance: Affect:

Effort: Level of Activity:

Unusual Behaviors:

Presenting Problem

Home

1.

2.

School

1.

2.

3.

4.

5.

Peers/Work

1.

2.

3.

4.

5.

Medication

Type:

Dosage:

Child's Name: _____

Date: _____

ADHD	ODD	CD

A. Inattention
  1. <a> <b>
  2. < >
  3. <a> <b>
  4. <a> <b> <c>
  5. < >
  6. < >
  7. < >
  8. <a> <b>
  9. <a> <b>
 	
B. Hyperactivity–Impulsivity
  1. <a> <b>
  2. <a> <b>
  3. < >
  4. <a> <b>
  5. < >
  6. <a> <b>
  7. < >
  8. <a> <b>
  9. <a> <b> <c>
	1. <a> <b>
	2. <a> <b>
	3. <a> <b> <c> <d>
	4. < >
	5. <a> <b>
	6. < >
	7. < >
	8. < >
		1. < >
		2. <a> <b>
		3. < >
		4. < >
		5. < >
		6. < >
		7. <a> <b>
		8. <a> <b>
		9. < >
		10. <a> <b>
		11. < >
		12. < >
		13. < >
		14. < >
		15. <a> <b>

Criteria If ≥6 in *A only*, then criteria met Inattentive < > If ≥6 in *B only*, then criteria met Hyperactive–Impulsive < > If ≥6 in A *and* ≥6 in B, then criteria met Combined < >	**Criteria** If ≥4, then criteria met ODD < >	**Criteria** If ≥3, then criteria met CD < >

Duration
1. _____ (years old)
2. < > _____ (years old)
3. < > _____ (months)
 	
  * DUR met for ADHD < >
	Duration
	1. _____ (years old)
	2. < > _____ (years old)
	3. < > _____ (months)
	
	  * DUR met for ODD < >
		Duration
		1. _____ (years old)
		2. < > _____ (years old)
		3. < > _____ (months)
		
		  * DUR met for CD < >

Impairment 1. < > home 2. < > school 3. < > peers	**Impairment** 1. < > home 2. < > school 3. < > peers	**Impairment** 1. < > home 2. < > school 3. < > peers
		Type Childhood Onset < > Adolescent Onset < > Mild < > Moderate < > Severe < >

SUB AB	PHO	SOCIAL PHO

1. < >
                 <a>_____
                 <b>_____
                 <c>_____
 	
      _____
2. < > _____
3. < > _____
4. < > _____
	1. _____
	   _____
	   _____
	2. <a> <b>
	3. <a> <b>
	4. <ai> <aii> <aiii> <aiv> <b>
	5. <a> <b>
		1. <a> <b>
		2. < >
		3. <a> <b>
		4. <ai> <aii> <aiii> <aiv> <b>
		5. < >

Duration
1. _____ (years old)
2. < > _____ (years old)
     _____ (months)
 	
   * DUR met for SUB AB < >
	Criteria
	   If 1–4, then criteria met
	         PHO < >
		Criteria
		   If 1–4, then criteria met
		     SOCIAL PHO < >

	Duration
	1. _____ (years old)
	2. < > _____ (years old)
	3. < > _____ (months)
	
	   * DUR met for PHO < >
		Duration
		1. _____ (years old)
		2. < > _____ (years old)
		3. < > _____ (months)
		
		   *DUR met for SOCIAL PHO < >

Impairment 1. <a> <b> 2. < > 3. <a> <b> 4. < >	**Impairment** 1. < > home 2. < > school 3. < > peers	**Impairment** 1. < > home 2. < > school 3. < > peers

Criteria
  If any use (Q1–4) and any
  impairment (1–4), then criteria
     met SUB AB < >
 	
Type(s) _____
_____
_____
_____
	Type(s)
	Animal < >
	Natural Environment < >
	Blood–Injection–Injury < >
	Situational < >
	Other _____ < >	

SEP ANX	GEN ANX	OCD

1. <a> <b>
2. <a> <b>
3. < >
4. <a> <b>
5. <a> <b>
6. <a> <b>
7. <a> <b>
8. <a> <b>
	1. < > _____
	_____
	_____
	_____
	_____
	2. <a> <b>
	3. <a> <b> <c> <d> <e> <f>
		A. Compulsions
		  1. < > _____
		  2. <a> _____
		    <b>
		  3. < >
		
		B. Obsessions
		  1. <a> _____
		    <b> _____
		    <c> _____
		  2. <a> <b> <c>
		  3. < >
		
		C. Interference
		  1. <a> <b> <c>

Criteria
  If ≥3, then criteria met
  SEP ANX < >
	Criteria
	  If 1–3, then criteria met
	  GEN ANX < >
		Criteria
		  If A1, A2, & C,
		  then criteria met
		  Compulsions < >
		
		  If B1, B2, & C,
		  then criteria met
		  Obsessions < >
		
		  If Compulsions +
		  and/or Obsessions +,
		  then criteria met
		  OCD < >

Duration
1. _____ (years old)
2. < > _____ (years old)
3. < > _____ (weeks)
 	
  *DUR met for SEP ANX < >
	Duration
	1. _____ (years old)
	2. < > _____ (years old)
	3. < > _____ (months)
	
	  *DUR met for GEN ANX < >
		Duration
		1. _____ (years old)
		2. < > _____ (years old)
		    _____ (months)
		
		  *DUR met for OCD < >

Impairment 1. < > home 2. < > school 3. < > peers	**Impairment** 1. < > home 2. < > school 3. < > peers	**Impairment** 1. < > home 2. < > school 3. < > peers

STRESS (ASD/PTSD)	ANO	BUL

A. Exposure
  1. \<a> \<b> _____
  2. \<a> \<b> \<c> \<d> \<e>
  3. \< > _____
B. Dissociation
  1. \<a> \<b> \<c> \<d>
  2. \< >
  3. \< >
  4. \< >
  5. \< >
C. Reexperiencing
  1. \<a> \<b> \<c>
  2. \<a> \<b>
  3. \<a> \<b>
  4. \<a> \<b>
  5. \< >
D. Avoidance
  1. \<a> \<b>
  2. \<a> \<b> \<c>
  3. \< >
  4. \<a> \<b>
  5. \<a> \<b>
  6. \<a> \<b>
  7. \<a> \<b>
E. Hyperarousal
  1. \<a> \<b>
  2. \<a> \<b>
  3. \< >
  4. \< >
  5. \< >
	1. \<a> \<b>
	2. \<a>
	  ht: _____
	  wt: _____
	  \<b>
	  ht: _____
	  wt: _____
	3. \<a> \<b> \<c>
	4. \<a> \<b> \<c>
	5. \< >
		1. \< > _____
		_____
		_
		2. \<a> \<b> \<c> \<d>
		3. \<a> \<b> \<c> \<d>
		4. \<a> \<b>

Criteria If A1 & A2, ≥3 in B, ≥1 in C, ≥3 in D, and ≥2 in E, then criteria met ASD \< > If A1 & A2, ≥1 in C, ≥3 in D, and ≥2 in E, then criteria met PTSD \< >	**Criteria** If 1–4 (&5 for pubescent girls), then criteria met ANO \< >	**Criteria** If 1–4, then criteria met BUL \< >

Duration
1. _____ (years old)
2. \< > _____ (years old)
3. a. \< > _____ (weeks)
  b. \< >
  c. \< > _____ (days)
4. \< > _____ (months)
    *DUR met for ASD \< >
    *DUR met for PTSD \< >
	Duration
	1. _____ (years old)
	2. \< > _____ (years old)
	3. \< > _____ (months)
	
	    *DUR met for ANO \< >
		Duration
		1. _____ (years old)
		2. \< > _____ (years old)
		3. a. \< > ____ (#/week)
		  b. \< > _____ (months)
		
		    *DUR met for BUL \< >

Impairment 1. \< > home 2. \< > school 3. \< > peers	**Impairment** 1. \< > home 2. \< > school 3. \< > peers	**Impairment** 1. \< > home 2. \< > school 3. \< > peers
Type (PTSD) Acute \< > Regular Onset \< > Chronic \< > Delayed Onset \< >		

DEP/DYS (MDD/DD)	DEP/DYS (MDD/DD)	MAN/HYPOMAN

A. Dysphoric Mood
  1. \<a> \<b> \<c>
  2. \<a> \<bi> \<bii> \<biii>
    \<c> \<d>
 	
B. Loss of Interest
  1. \<a> \<b>
  2. \<a> \<b> \<c>
 	
C. Appetite Changes
  1. \<a> \<b> \<c>
  2. \<a> \<b>
 	
D. Sleep Changes
    Bedtime: _____
    Wakeup: _____
  1. \<a> \<b> \<c>
  2. \<a> \<b>
 	
E. Psychomotor Changes
  1. \<a> \<b> \<c> \<d>
  2. \<a> \<b>
 	
F. Low Energy
  1. \<a> \<b> \<c> \<d>
 	
G. Guilt
  1. \<a> \<b> \<c> \<d>
  2. \<a> \<b>
 	
H. Impaired Concentration
  1. \<a> \<b> \<c> \<d> \<e>
  2. \< >
 	
I. Hopelessness
  1. \<a> \<b> \<c>
 	
J. Morbid/Suicidal Thoughts
  1. \<a> \<b>
  2. \<a> \<b> \<c> \<d> \<e>
 	
_____
_____
_____
_____
_____
		A. Elevated Mood
		  1. \<a> _____
		    \<b> _____
		    \<c> _____
		  2. \< > _____
		
		B. Other Symptoms
		  1. \<a> _____
		    \<b>
		  2. \<a> \<b> \<c> _____
		  3. \<a> \<b> \<c> \<d>
		  4. \<a> \<b> \<c>
		  5. \< >
		  6. \<a> \<b> \<c> \<d> \<e>
		  7. \<a> \<b> \<c> \<d>
		
		C. Interference
		  1. \< >
		  2. \< >

	Criteria If A &/or B & ≥5 of A–H or J, then criteria met MDD \< > If A & ≥2 of C, D, F, G, H, or I, then criteria met DD \< >	**Criteria** If A1(a, b, & c) + ≥3 in B + ≥1 in C *or* A2 + ≥4 in B + ≥1 in C, then criteria met MAN \< > If A1(a, b, & c) + ≥3 in B + none in C *or* A2 + ≥4 in B + none in C, then criteria met HYPOMAN \< >

	Duration
	1. _____ (years old)
	2. \< > _____ (years old)
	3. MDD \< > _____ (weeks)
	   DD \< > _____ (months)
	
	  *DUR met for MDD \< >
	  *DUR met for DD \< >
		Duration
		1. _____ (years old)
		2. \< > _____ (years old)
		3. MAN \< > _____ (weeks)
		   HYPO \< > _____ (days)
		
		  *DUR met for MAN \< >
		  *DUR met for HYPOMAN \< >

	Impairment 1. \< > home 2. \< > school 3. \< > peers	**Impairment** 1. \< > home 2. \< > school 3. \< > peers

ENU	SCZ/PSY	STRESSORS

1. < >
2. <a> <b>
3. <a> <b>
 	
Criteria
If 1, ≥1 in 2, 3a, and 3b,
then criteria met
ENU < >
 	
Duration
1. _____ (years old)
2. < > _____ (years old)
3. <a> _____ (x/week)
   <b> _____ (months)
 	
  *DUR met for ENU < >
 	
Impairment
1. < > home
2. < > school
3. < > peers
 	
Type
Nocturnal   < >
Diurnal   < >
Both   < >
 	
ENC
 	
1. < >
2. < >
 	
Criteria
If both 1 & 2, then criteria met
ENC < >
 	
Duration
1. _____ (years old)
2. < > _____ (years old)
3. <a> _____ (x/month)
   <b> _____ (months)
 	
  *DUR met for ENC < >
 	
Impairment
1. < > home
2. < > school
3. < > peers
	A. Psychotic Symptoms
	  1. <a> <b> <c> <d> <e>
	  2. <a> <b> <c> <d> <e> <f>
	  3. < >
	  4. < >
	  5. < >
	
	B. Interference
	  1. < >
	  2. < >
	  3. < >
	
	Criteria
	If ≥2 in A and ≥1 in B,
	then criteria met
	SCZ < >
	
	If ≥1 in A, then criteria met
	PSY < >
	
	Duration
	1. _____ (years old)
	2. < > _____ (years old)
	3. < > _____ (months)
	
	  *DUR met for SCZ < >
	  *DUR met for PSY < >
	
	Impairment
	1. < > home
	2. < > school
	3. < > peers
		A. Child Abuse/Neglect
		1. <a> <b> <c>
		2. <a> <b> <c> <d>
		3. <a> <b> <c> <d>
		4. < >
		5. < >
		
		Duration
		1. _____
		2. < > _____
		3. _____
		4. _____
		5. < >
		
		B. Other Stressors
		1. <a> <b> <c> <d> <e>
		2. < >
		3. <a> <b>
		4. <a> <b> <c>
		5. <a> <b>
		6. <a> <b>
		7. <a> _____
		     <b>
		8. <a> <b> <c> <d>
		9. < > _____
		    _____
		    _____
		10. < > _____
		11. < > _____
		    _____
		    _____

Child's Number: _____ Date: _____

Child's Name: _____ Time Started: _____

Date of Birth: _____ Age: _____ Time Ended: _____

Race: _____ Sex: _____ Interviewer: _____

Setting (circle one):   Inpatient,   Outpatient,   School,   Other Research Setting: _____

	Disorder	Symptoms	Diagnosis	Duration	Clinician's Diagnosis
ADHD	**Attention-Deficit/Hyperactivity Disorder** *Type:* Inattentive, Hyperactive–Impulsive, Combined	<>	<>	<>	Axis I
ODD	**Oppositional Defiant Disorder**	<>	<>	<>	
CD	**Conduct Disorder** *Onset:* Childhood, Adolescent *Severity:* Mild, Moderate, Severe	<>	<>	<>	
SUBAB	**Substance Abuse** *Substance(s):* _____	<>	<>	<>	
PHO	**Specific Phobia** *Type:* _____	<>	<>	<>	Axis II
SOCPHO	**Social Phobia**	<>	<>	<>	
SEPANX	**Separation Anxiety Disorder**	<>	<>	<>	Axis III
GENANX	**General Anxiety Disorder**	<>	<>	<>	
OCD	**Obsessive-Compulsive Disorder**	<>	<>	<>	
PTSD	**Posttraumatic Stress Disorder** *Type:* Acute, Chronic *Onset:* Regular, Delayed	<>	<>	<>	Axis IV
ASD	**Acute Stress Disorder**	<>	<>	<>	
ANO	**Anorexia**	<>	<>	<>	Axis V
BUL	**Bulimia**	<>	<>	<>	current:
DEP	**Major Depressive Disorder**	<>	<>	<>	past year:
DYS	**Dysthymic Disorder**	<>	<>	<>	
MAN	**Mania**	<>	<>	<>	
HYPOMAN	**Hypomania**	<>	<>	<>	
ENU	**Enuresis** *Type:* Nocturnal, Diurnal, Both	<>	<>	<>	
ENC	**Encopresis**	<>	<>	<>	
SCZ	**Schizophrenia**	<>	<>	<>	
PSY	**Psychosis**	<>	<>	<>	

Psychosocial Stressors:

Other Stressors:

Behavioral Observations

Appearance: Affect:

Effort: Level of Activity:

Unusual Behaviors:

Presenting Problem

Home

1.

2.

School

1.

2.

3.

4.

5.

Peers/Work

1.

2.

3.

4.

5.

Medication

Type:

Dosage:

Child's Name: _____

Date: _____

ADHD	ODD	CD

A. Inattention
   1. \<a> \<b>
   2. \< >
   3. \<a> \<b>
   4. \<a> \<b> \<c>
   5. \< >
   6. \< >
   7. \< >
   8. \<a> \<b>
   9. \<a> \<b>
 	
B. Hyperactivity–Impulsivity
   1. \<a> \<b>
   2. \<a> \<b>
   3. \< >
   4. \<a> \<b>
   5. \< >
   6. \<a> \<b>
   7. \< >
   8. \<a> \<b>
   9. \<a> \<b> \<c>
	1. \<a> \<b>
	2. \<a> \<b>
	3. \<a> \<b> \<c> \<d>
	4. \< >
	5. \<a> \<b>
	6. \< >
	7. \< >
	8. \< >
		1. \< >
		2. \<a> \<b>
		3. \< >
		4. \< >
		5. \< >
		6. \< >
		7. \<a> \<b>
		8. \<a> \<b>
		9. \< >
		10. \<a> \<b>
		11. \< >
		12. \< >
		13. \< >
		14. \< >
		15. \<a> \<b>

Criteria If ≥6 in *A only*, then criteria met Inattentive \< > If ≥6 in *B only*, then criteria met Hyperactive–Impulsive \< > If ≥6 in A *and* ≥6 in B, then criteria met Combined \< >	**Criteria** If ≥4, then criteria met ODD \< >	**Criteria** If ≥3, then criteria met CD \< >

Duration
1. _____ (years old)
2. \< > _____ (years old)
3. \< > _____ (months)
 	
   * DUR met for ADHD \< >
	Duration
	1. _____ (years old)
	2. \< > _____ (years old)
	3. \< > _____ (months)
	
	   * DUR met for ODD \< >
		Duration
		1. _____ (years old)
		2. \< > _____ (years old)
		3. \< > _____ (months)
		
		   * DUR met for CD \< >

Impairment 1. \< > home 2. \< > school 3. \< > peers	**Impairment** 1. \< > home 2. \< > school 3. \< > peers	**Impairment** 1. \< > home 2. \< > school 3. \< > peers
		Type Childhood Onset \< > Adolescent Onset \< > Mild \< > Moderate \< > Severe \< >

SUB AB	PHO	SOCIAL PHO

1. < >
     <a>_____
     <b>_____
     <c>_____
 	
     _____
 2. < > _____
 3. < > _____
 4. < > _____
	1. _____
	     _____
	     _____
	 2. <a> <b>
	 3. <a> <b>
	 4. <ai> <aii> <aiii> <aiv> <b>
	 5. <a> <b>
		1. <a> <b>
		 2. < >
		 3. <a> <b>
		 4. <ai> <aii> <aiii> <aiv> <b>
		 5. < >

SUB AB — Duration

Duration
1. _____ (years old)
2. < > _____ (years old)
    _____ (months)

    * DUR met for SUB AB < >

PHO — Criteria

Criteria
    If 1–4, then criteria met
        PHO < >

SOCIAL PHO — Criteria

Criteria
    If 1–4, then criteria met
        SOCIAL PHO < >

PHO — Duration

Duration
1. _____ (years old)
2. < > _____ (years old)
3. < > _____ (months)

    * DUR met for PHO < >

SOCIAL PHO — Duration

Duration
1. _____ (years old)
2. < > _____ (years old)
3. < > _____ (months)

    *DUR met for SOCIAL PHO < >

SUB AB — Impairment

Impairment
1. <a> <b>
2. < >
3. <a> <b>
4. < >

PHO — Impairment

Impairment
1. < > home
2. < > school
3. < > peers

SOCIAL PHO — Impairment

Impairment
1. < > home
2. < > school
3. < > peers

SUB AB — Criteria

Criteria
    If any use (Q1–4) and any
    impairment (1–4), then criteria
        met SUB AB < >

Type(s) _____
_____
_____
_____

PHO — Type(s)

Type(s)
Animal   < >
Natural Environment   < >
Blood–Injection–Injury   < >
Situational   < >
Other _____   < >

SEP ANX	GEN ANX	OCD

1. \<a\> \<b\>
 2. \<a\> \<b\>
 3. \< \>
 4. \<a\> \<b\>
 5. \<a\> \<b\>
 6. \<a\> \<b\>
 7. \<a\> \<b\>
 8. \<a\> \<b\>
	1. \< \> _____
	 _____
	 _____
	 _____
	 _____
	 2. \<a\> \<b\>
	 3. \<a\> \<b\> \<c\> \<d\> \<e\> \<f\>
		A. Compulsions
		   1. \< \> _____
		   2. \<a\> _____
		     \<b\>
		   3. \< \>
		
		 B. Obsessions
		   1. \<a\> _____
		     \<b\> _____
		     \<c\> _____
		   2. \<a\> \<b\> \<c\>
		   3. \< \>
		
		 C. Interference
		   1. \<a\> \<b\> \<c\>

Criteria If ≥3, then criteria met SEP ANX \< \>	**Criteria** If 1–3, then criteria met GEN ANX \< \>	**Criteria** If A1, A2, & C, then criteria met Compulsions \< \> If B1, B2, & C, then criteria met Obsessions \< \> If Compulsions + and/or Obsessions +, then criteria met OCD \< \>
Duration 1. _____ (years old) 2. \< \> _____ (years old) 3. \< \> _____ (weeks) *DUR met for SEP ANX \< \>	**Duration** 1. _____ (years old) 2. \< \> _____ (years old) 3. \< \> _____ (months) *DUR met for GEN ANX \< \>	**Duration** 1. _____ (years old) 2. \< \> _____ (years old) _____ (months) *DUR met for OCD \< \>
Impairment 1. \< \> home 2. \< \> school 3. \< \> peers	**Impairment** 1. \< \> home 2. \< \> school 3. \< \> peers	**Impairment** 1. \< \> home 2. \< \> school 3. \< \> peers

STRESS (ASD/PTSD)	ANO	BUL

A. Exposure
  1. \<a> \<b> _____
  2. \<a> \<b> \<c> \<d> \<e>
  3. \< > _____
B. Dissociation
  1. \<a> \<b> \<c> \<d>
  2. \< >
  3. \< >
  4. \< >
  5. \< >
C. Reexperiencing
  1. \<a> \<b> \<c>
  2. \<a> \<b>
  3. \<a> \<b>
  4. \<a> \<b>
  5. \< >
D. Avoidance
  1. \<a> \<b>
  2. \<a> \<b> \<c>
  3. \< >
  4. \<a> \<b>
  5. \<a> \<b>
  6. \<a> \<b>
  7. \<a> \<b>
E. Hyperarousal
  1. \<a> \<b>
  2. \<a> \<b>
  3. \< >
  4. \< >
  5. \< >
	1. \<a> \<b>
	2. \<a>
	  ht: _____
	  wt: _____
	  \<b>
	  ht: _____
	  wt: _____
	3. \<a> \<b> \<c>
	4. \<a> \<b> \<c>
	5. \< >
		1. \< > _____
		_____
		 –
		2. \<a> \<b> \<c> \<d>
		3. \<a> \<b> \<c> \<d>
		4. \<a> \<b>

Criteria If A1 & A2, ≥3 in B, ≥1 in C, ≥3 in D, and ≥2 in E, then criteria met ASD \< > If A1 & A2, ≥1 in C, ≥3 in D, and ≥2 in E, then criteria met PTSD \< >	**Criteria** If 1–4 (&5 for pubescent girls), then criteria met ANO \< >	**Criteria** If 1–4, then criteria met BUL \< >

Duration
1. _____ (years old)
2. \< > _____ (years old)
3. a. \< > _____ (weeks)
   b. \< >
   c. \< > _____ (days)
4. \< > _____ (months)
    *DUR met for ASD \< >
    *DUR met for PTSD \< >
	Duration
	1. _____ (years old)
	2. \< > _____ (years old)
	3. \< > _____ (months)
	
	   *DUR met for ANO \< >
		Duration
		1. _____ (years old)
		2. \< > _____ (years old)
		3. a. \< > _____ (#/week)
		   b. \< > _____ (months)
		
		   *DUR met for BUL \< >

Impairment 1. \< > home 2. \< > school 3. \< > peers	**Impairment** 1. \< > home 2. \< > school 3. \< > peers	**Impairment** 1. \< > home 2. \< > school 3. \< > peers
Type (PTSD) Acute \< > Regular Onset \< > Chronic \< > Delayed Onset \< >		

DEP/DYS (MDD/DD)	DEP/DYS (MDD/DD)	MAN/HYPOMAN

A. Dysphoric Mood
  1. \<a> \<b> \<c>
  2. \<a> \<bi> \<bii> \<biii>
    \<c> \<d>
 	
B. Loss of Interest
  1. \<a> \<b>
  2. \<a> \<b> \<c>
 	
C. Appetite Changes
  1. \<a> \<b> \<c>
  2. \<a> \<b>
 	
D. Sleep Changes
    Bedtime: _____
    Wakeup: _____
  1. \<a> \<b> \<c>
  2. \<a> \<b>
 	
E. Psychomotor Changes
  1. \<a> \<b> \<c> \<d>
  2. \<a> \<b>
 	
F. Low Energy
  1. \<a> \<b> \<c> \<d>
 	
G. Guilt
  1. \<a> \<b> \<c> \<d>
  2. \<a> \<b>
 	
H. Impaired Concentration
  1. \<a> \<b> \<c> \<d> \<e>
  2. \< >
 	
I. Hopelessness
  1. \<a> \<b> \<c>
 	
J. Morbid/Suicidal Thoughts
  1. \<a> \<b>
  2. \<a> \<b> \<c> \<d> \<e>
 	
_____
_____
_____
_____
_____
		A. Elevated Mood
		  1. \<a> _____
		    \<b> _____
		    \<c> _____
		  2. \< > _____
		
		B. Other Symptoms
		  1. \<a> _____
		    \<b>
		  2. \<a> \<b> \<c> _____
		  3. \<a> \<b> \<c> \<d>
		  4. \<a> \<b> \<c>
		  5. \< >
		  6. \<a> \<b> \<c> \<d> \<e>
		  7. \<a> \<b> \<c> \<d>
		
		C. Interference
		  1. \< >
		  2. \< >

	Criteria If A &/or B & ≥5 of A–H or J, then criteria met MDD \< > If A & ≥2 of C, D, F, G, H, or I, then criteria met DD \< >	**Criteria** If A1(a, b, & c) + ≥3 in B + ≥1 in C *or* A2 + ≥4 in B + ≥1 in C, then criteria met MAN \< > If A1(a, b, & c) + ≥3 in B + none in C *or* A2 + ≥4 in B + none in C, then criteria met HYPOMAN \< >

	Duration
	1. _____ (years old)
	2. \< > _____ (years old)
	3. MDD \< > _____ (weeks)
	    DD \< > _____ (months)
	
	   *DUR met for MDD \< >
	   *DUR met for DD \< >
		Duration
		1. _____ (years old)
		2. \< > _____ (years old)
		3. MAN \< > _____ (weeks)
		    HYPO \< > _____ (days)
		
		   *DUR met for MAN \< >
		   *DUR met for HYPOMAN \< >

	Impairment 1. \< > home 2. \< > school 3. \< > peers	**Impairment** 1. \< > home 2. \< > school 3. \< > peers

ENU	SCZ/PSY	STRESSORS

1. < >
2. <a> <b>
3. <a> <b>
	A. Psychotic Symptoms
	  1. <a> <b> <c> <d> <e>
	  2. <a> <b> <c> <d> <e> <f>
	  3. < >
	  4. < >
	  5. < >
		A. Child Abuse/Neglect
		1. <a> <b> <c>
		2. <a> <b> <c> <d>
		3. <a> <b> <c> <d>
		4. < >
		5. < >

Criteria
   If 1, ≥1 in 2, 3a, and 3b,
     then criteria met
       ENU < >
	B. Interference
	  1. < >
	  2. < >
	  3. < >
		Duration
		1. _____
		2. < > _____
		3. _____
		4. _____
		5. < >

Duration
1. _____ (years old)
2. < > _____ (years old)
3. <a> _____ (x/week)
   <b> _____ (months)
 	
   *DUR met for ENU < >
	Criteria
	   If ≥2 in A and ≥1 in B,
	     then criteria met
	       SCZ < >
	
	   If ≥1 in A, then criteria met
	       PSY < >
		B. Other Stressors
		  1. <a> <b> <c> <d> <e>
		  2. < >
		  3. <a> <b>
		  4. <a> <b> <c>
		  5. <a> <b>
		  6. <a> <b>
		  7. <a> _____
		       <b>
		  8. <a> <b> <c> <d>
		  9. < > _____

Impairment
1. < > home
2. < > school
3. < > peers
	Duration
	1. _____ (years old)
	2. < > _____ (years old)
	3. < > _____ (months)
	
	   *DUR met for SCZ < >
	   *DUR met for PSY < >
		_____
		_____
		10. < >
		11. < > _____

Type Nocturnal < > Diurnal < > Both < >	**Impairment** 1. < > home 2. < > school 3. < > peers	_____ _____
ENC		
1. < > 2. < >		
Criteria If both 1 & 2, then criteria met ENC < >		
Duration 1. _____ (years old) 2. < > _____ (years old) 3. <a> _____ (x/month) <b> _____ (months) *DUR met for ENC < >		
Impairment 1. < > home 2. < > school 3. < > peers		

ChIPS Scoring Form
Profile Sheet

Child's Number: _____   Date: _____

Child's Name: _____   Time Started: _____

Date of Birth: _____ Age: _____   Time Ended: _____

Race: _____ Sex: _____   Interviewer: _____

Setting (circle one):   Inpatient,   Outpatient,   School,   Other Research Setting: _____

	Disorder	Symptoms	Diagnosis	Duration	Clinician's Diagnosis
ADHD	Attention-Deficit/Hyperactivity Disorder	<>	<>	<>	Axis I
	Type: Inattentive, Hyperactive–Impulsive, Combined				
ODD	Oppositional Defiant Disorder	<>	<>	<>	
CD	Conduct Disorder	<>	<>	<>	
	Onset: Childhood, Adolescent				
	Severity: Mild, Moderate, Severe				
SUBAB	Substance Abuse	<>	<>	<>	
	Substance(s): _____				
PHO	Specific Phobia	<>	<>	<>	Axis II
	Type: _____				
SOCPHO	Social Phobia	<>	<>	<>	
SEPANX	Separation Anxiety Disorder	<>	<>	<>	Axis III
GENANX	General Anxiety Disorder	<>	<>	<>	
OCD	Obsessive-Compulsive Disorder	<>	<>	<>	
PTSD	Posttraumatic Stress Disorder	<>	<>	<>	Axis IV
	Type: Acute, Chronic				
	Onset: Regular, Delayed				
ASD	Acute Stress Disorder	<>	<>	<>	
ANO	Anorexia	<>	<>	<>	Axis V
BUL	Bulimia	<>	<>	<>	current:
DEP	Major Depressive Disorder	<>	<>	<>	past year:
DYS	Dysthymic Disorder	<>	<>	<>	
MAN	Mania	<>	<>	<>	
HYPOMAN	Hypomania	<>	<>	<>	
ENU	Enuresis	<>	<>	<>	
	Type: Nocturnal, Diurnal, Both				
ENC	Encopresis	<>	<>	<>	
SCZ	Schizophrenia	<>	<>	<>	
PSY	Psychosis	<>	<>	<>	

Psychosocial Stressors:

Other Stressors:

Behavioral Observations

Appearance: Affect:

Effort: Level of Activity:

Unusual Behaviors:

Presenting Problem

Home

1.

2.

School

1.

2.

3.

4.

5.

Peers/Work

1.

2.

3.

4.

5.

Medication

Type:

Dosage:

Child's Name: _____

Date: _____

ADHD	ODD	CD

A. Inattention
  1. \<a> \<b>
  2. \< >
  3. \<a> \<b>
  4. \<a> \<b> \<c>
  5. \< >
  6. \< >
  7. \< >
  8. \<a> \<b>
  9. \<a> \<b>
 	
B. Hyperactivity–Impulsivity
  1. \<a> \<b>
  2. \<a> \<b>
  3. \< >
  4. \<a> \<b>
  5. \< >
  6. \<a> \<b>
  7. \< >
  8. \<a> \<b>
  9. \<a> \<b> \<c>
	1. \<a> \<b>
	2. \<a> \<b>
	3. \<a> \<b> \<c> \<d>
	4. \< >
	5. \<a> \<b>
	6. \< >
	7. \< >
	8. \< >
		1. \< >
		2. \<a> \<b>
		3. \< >
		4. \< >
		5. \< >
		6. \< >
		7. \<a> \<b>
		8. \<a> \<b>
		9. \< >
		10. \<a> \<b>
		11. \< >
		12. \< >
		13. \< >
		14. \< >
		15. \<a> \<b>

Criteria If ≥6 in *A only*, then criteria met Inattentive \< > If ≥6 in *B only*, then criteria met Hyperactive–Impulsive \< > If ≥6 in A *and* ≥6 in B, then criteria met Combined \< >	**Criteria** If ≥4, then criteria met ODD \< >	**Criteria** If ≥3, then criteria met CD \< >

Duration
1. _____ (years old)
2. \< > _____ (years old)
3. \< > _____ (months)
 	
  * DUR met for ADHD \< >
	Duration
	1. _____ (years old)
	2. \< > _____ (years old)
	3. \< > _____ (months)
	
	  * DUR met for ODD \< >
		Duration
		1. _____ (years old)
		2. \< > _____ (years old)
		3. \< > _____ (months)
		
		  * DUR met for CD \< >

Impairment 1. \< > home 2. \< > school 3. \< > peers	**Impairment** 1. \< > home 2. \< > school 3. \< > peers	**Impairment** 1. \< > home 2. \< > school 3. \< > peers
		Type Childhood Onset \< > Adolescent Onset \< > Mild \< > Moderate \< > Severe \< >

SUB AB	PHO	SOCIAL PHO

1. < >
    <a>_____
    <b>_____
    <c>_____
 	
    _____
2. < > _____
3. < > _____
4. < > _____
	1. _____
	   _____
	   _____
	2. <a> <b>
	3. <a> <b>
	4. <ai> <aii> <aiii> <aiv> <b>
	5. <a> <b>
		1. <a> <b>
		2. < >
		3. <a> <b>
		4. <ai> <aii> <aiii> <aiv> <b>
		5. < >

Duration
1. _____ (years old)
2. < > _____ (years old)
    _____ (months)
 	
  * DUR met for SUB AB < >
	Criteria
	  If 1–4, then criteria met
	    PHO < >
		Criteria
		  If 1–4, then criteria met
		   SOCIAL PHO < >

	Duration 1. _____ (years old) 2. < > _____ (years old) 3. < > _____ (months) * DUR met for PHO < >	**Duration** 1. _____ (years old) 2. < > _____ (years old) 3. < > _____ (months) *DUR met for SOCIAL PHO < >
Impairment 1. <a> <b> 2. < > 3. <a> <b> 4. < >	**Impairment** 1. < > home 2. < > school 3. < > peers	**Impairment** 1. < > home 2. < > school 3. < > peers

Criteria
  If any use (Q1–4) and any
  impairment (1–4), then criteria
    met SUB AB < >
 	
Type(s) _____
_____
_____
_____
	Type(s)
	Animal < >
	Natural Environment < >
	Blood–Injection–Injury < >
	Situational < >
	Other _____ < >	

SEP ANX	GEN ANX	OCD

1. <a> <b>
 2. <a> <b>
 3. < >
 4. <a> <b>
 5. <a> <b>
 6. <a> <b>
 7. <a> <b>
 8. <a> <b>
	1. < > _____
	 _____
	 _____
	 _____
	 _____
	 2. <a> <b>
	 3. <a> <b> <c> <d> <e> <f>
		A. Compulsions
		   1. < > _____
		   2. <a> _____
		      <b>
		   3. < >
		
		 B. Obsessions
		   1. <a> _____
		      <b> _____
		      <c> _____
		   2. <a> <b> <c>
		   3. < >
		
		 C. Interference
		   1. <a> <b> <c>

Criteria If ≥3, then criteria met SEP ANX < >	**Criteria** If 1–3, then criteria met GEN ANX < >	**Criteria** If A1, A2, & C, then criteria met Compulsions < > If B1, B2, & C, then criteria met Obsessions < > If Compulsions + and/or Obsessions +, then criteria met OCD < >
Duration 1. _____ (years old) 2. < > _____ (years old) 3. < > _____ (weeks) *DUR met for SEP ANX < >	**Duration** 1. _____ (years old) 2. < > _____ (years old) 3. < > _____ (months) *DUR met for GEN ANX < >	**Duration** 1. _____ (years old) 2. < > _____ (years old) _____ (months) *DUR met for OCD < >
Impairment 1. < > home 2. < > school 3. < > peers	**Impairment** 1. < > home 2. < > school 3. < > peers	**Impairment** 1. < > home 2. < > school 3. < > peers

STRESS (ASD/PTSD)	ANO	BUL

A. Exposure
  1. \<a> \<b> _____
  2. \<a> \<b> \<c> \<d> \<e>
  3. \< > _____
B. Dissociation
  1. \<a> \<b> \<c> \<d>
  2. \< >
  3. \< >
  4. \< >
  5. \< >
C. Reexperiencing
  1. \<a> \<b> \<c>
  2. \<a> \<b>
  3. \<a> \<b>
  4. \<a> \<b>
  5. \< >
D. Avoidance
  1. \<a> \<b>
  2. \<a> \<b> \<c>
  3. \< >
  4. \<a> \<b>
  5. \<a> \<b>
  6. \<a> \<b>
  7. \<a> \<b>
E. Hyperarousal
  1. \<a> \<b>
  2. \<a> \<b>
  3. \< >
  4. \< >
  5. \< >
	1. \<a> \<b>
	2. \<a>
	  ht: _____
	  wt: _____
	  \<b>
	  ht: _____
	  wt: _____
	3. \<a> \<b> \<c>
	4. \<a> \<b> \<c>
	5. \< >
		1. \< > _____
		_____
		_
		2. \<a> \<b> \<c> \<d>
		3. \<a> \<b> \<c> \<d>
		4. \<a> \<b>

Criteria If A1 *&* A2, ≥3 in B, ≥1 in C, ≥3 in D, and ≥2 in E, then criteria met ASD \< > If A1 *&* A2, ≥1 in C, ≥3 in D, and ≥2 in E, then criteria met PTSD \< >	**Criteria** If 1–4 (&5 for pubescent girls), then criteria met ANO \< >	**Criteria** If 1–4, then criteria met BUL \< >

Duration
1. _____ (years old)
2. \< > _____ (years old)
3. a. \< > _____ (weeks)
   b. \< >
   c. \< > _____ (days)
4. \< > _____ (months)
    *DUR met for ASD \< >
    *DUR met for PTSD \< >
	Duration
	1. _____ (years old)
	2. \< > _____ (years old)
	3. \< > _____ (months)
	
	  *DUR met for ANO \< >
		Duration
		1. _____ (years old)
		2. \< > _____ (years old)
		3. a. \< > _____ (#/week)
		   b. \< > _____ (months)
		
		  *DUR met for BUL \< >

Impairment 1. \< > home 2. \< > school 3. \< > peers	**Impairment** 1. \< > home 2. \< > school 3. \< > peers	**Impairment** 1. \< > home 2. \< > school 3. \< > peers
Type (PTSD) Acute \< > Regular Onset \< > Chronic \< > Delayed Onset \< >		

DEP/DYS (MDD/DD)	DEP/DYS (MDD/DD)	MAN/HYPOMAN

A. Dysphoric Mood
  1. \<a\> \<b\> \<c\>
  2. \<a\> \<bi\> \<bii\> \<biii\>
    \<c\> \<d\>
 	
B. Loss of Interest
  1. \<a\> \<b\>
  2. \<a\> \<b\> \<c\>
 	
C. Appetite Changes
  1. \<a\> \<b\> \<c\>
  2. \<a\> \<b\>
 	
D. Sleep Changes
    Bedtime: _____
    Wakeup: _____
  1. \<a\> \<b\> \<c\>
  2. \<a\> \<b\>
 	
E. Psychomotor Changes
  1. \<a\> \<b\> \<c\> \<d\>
  2. \<a\> \<b\>
 	
F. Low Energy
  1. \<a\> \<b\> \<c\> \<d\>
 	
G. Guilt
  1. \<a\> \<b\> \<c\> \<d\>
  2. \<a\> \<b\>
 	
H. Impaired Concentration
  1. \<a\> \<b\> \<c\> \<d\> \<e\>
  2. \< \>
 	
I. Hopelessness
  1. \<a\> \<b\> \<c\>
 	
J. Morbid/Suicidal Thoughts
  1. \<a\> \<b\>
  2. \<a\> \<b\> \<c\> \<d\> \<e\>
 	
_____
_____
_____
_____
_____
		A. Elevated Mood
		  1. \<a\> _____
		    \<b\> _____
		    \<c\> _____
		  2. \< \> _____
		
		B. Other Symptoms
		  1. \<a\> _____
		    \<b\>
		  2. \<a\> \<b\> \<c\> _____
		  3. \<a\> \<b\> \<c\> \<d\>
		  4. \<a\> \<b\> \<c\>
		  5. \< \>
		  6. \<a\> \<b\> \<c\> \<d\> \<e\>
		  7. \<a\> \<b\> \<c\> \<d\>
		
		C. Interference
		  1. \< \>
		  2. \< \>

	Criteria If A &/or B & ≥5 of A–H or J, then criteria met MDD \< \> If A & ≥2 of C, D, F, G, H, or I, then criteria met DD \< \>	**Criteria** If A1(a, b, & c) + ≥3 in B + ≥1 in C *or* A2 + ≥4 in B + ≥1 in C, then criteria met MAN \< \> If A1(a, b, & c) + ≥3 in B + none in C *or* A2 + ≥4 in B + none in C, then criteria met HYPOMAN \< \>

	Duration
	1. _____ (years old)
	2. \< \> _____ (years old)
	3. MDD \< \> _____ (weeks)
	  DD \< \> _____ (months)
	
	  *DUR met for MDD \< \>
	  *DUR met for DD \< \>
		Duration
		1. _____ (years old)
		2. \< \> _____ (years old)
		3. MAN \< \> _____ (weeks)
		  HYPO \< \> _____ (days)
		
		  *DUR met for MAN \< \>
		  *DUR met for HYPOMAN \< \>

	Impairment 1. \< \> home 2. \< \> school 3. \< \> peers	**Impairment** 1. \< \> home 2. \< \> school 3. \< \> peers

ENU	SCZ/PSY	STRESSORS

1. < >
 2. \<a\> \<b\>
 3. \<a\> \<b\>
 	
 Criteria
     If 1, ≥1 in 2, 3a, and 3b,
       then criteria met
         ENU < >
 	
 Duration
 1. _____ (years old)
 2. < > _____ (years old)
 3. \<a\> _____ (x/week)
    \<b\> _____ (months)
 	
    *DUR met for ENU < >
 	
 Impairment
 1. < > home
 2. < > school
 3. < > peers
 	
 Type
 Nocturnal   < >
 Diurnal   < >
 Both   < >
	A. Psychotic Symptoms
	    1. \<a\> \<b\> \<c\> \<d\> \<e\>
	    2. \<a\> \<b\> \<c\> \<d\> \<e\> \<f\>
	    3. < >
	    4. < >
	    5. < >
	
	 B. Interference
	    1. < >
	    2. < >
	    3. < >
	
	 Criteria
	    If ≥2 in A and ≥1 in B,
	      then criteria met
	        SCZ < >
	
	    If ≥1 in A, then criteria met
	        PSY < >
	
	 Duration
	 1. _____ (years old)
	 2. < > _____ (years old)
	 3. < > _____ (months)
	
	    *DUR met for SCZ < >
	    *DUR met for PSY < >
	
	 Impairment
	 1. < > home
	 2. < > school
	 3. < > peers
		A. Child Abuse/Neglect
		 1. \<a\> \<b\> \<c\>
		 2. \<a\> \<b\> \<c\> \<d\>
		 3. \<a\> \<b\> \<c\> \<d\>
		 4. < >
		 5. < >
		
		 Duration
		 1. _____
		 2. < > _____
		 3. _____
		 4. _____
		 5. < >
		
		 B. Other Stressors
		    1. \<a\> \<b\> \<c\> \<d\> \<e\>
		    2. < >
		    3. \<a\> \<b\>
		    4. \<a\> \<b\> \<c\>
		    5. \<a\> \<b\>
		    6. \<a\> \<b\>
		    7. \<a\> _____
		        \<b\>
		    8. \<a\> \<b\> \<c\> \<d\>
		    9. < > _____
		        _____
		        _____
		   10. < >
		   11. < > _____
		        _____
		        _____

ENC

1. < >
2. < >

Criteria
If both 1 & 2, then criteria met
      ENC < >

Duration
1. _____ (years old)
2. < > _____ (years old)
3. \<a\> _____ (x/month)
   \<b\> _____ (months)

   *DUR met for ENC < >

Impairment
1. < > home
2. < > school
3. < > peers

Child's Number: _____   Date: _____

Child's Name: _____   Time Started: _____

Date of Birth: _____ Age: _____   Time Ended: _____

Race: _____ Sex: _____   Interviewer: _____

Setting (circle one):   Inpatient,   Outpatient,   School,   Other Research Setting: _____

	Disorder	Symptoms	Diagnosis	Duration	Clinician's Diagnosis
ADHD	Attention-Deficit/Hyperactivity Disorder	<>	<>	<>	Axis I
	Type: Inattentive, Hyperactive–Impulsive, Combined				
ODD	Oppositional Defiant Disorder	<>	<>	<>	
CD	Conduct Disorder	<>	<>	<>	
	Onset: Childhood, Adolescent				
	Severity: Mild, Moderate, Severe				
SUBAB	Substance Abuse	<>	<>	<>	
	Substance(s): _____				
PHO	Specific Phobia	<>	<>	<>	Axis II
	Type: _____				
SOCPHO	Social Phobia	<>	<>	<>	
SEPANX	Separation Anxiety Disorder	<>	<>	<>	Axis III
GENANX	General Anxiety Disorder	<>	<>	<>	
OCD	Obsessive-Compulsive Disorder	<>	<>	<>	
PTSD	Posttraumatic Stress Disorder	<>	<>	<>	Axis IV
	Type: Acute, Chronic				
	Onset: Regular, Delayed				
ASD	Acute Stress Disorder	<>	<>	<>	
ANO	Anorexia	<>	<>	<>	Axis V
BUL	Bulimia	<>	<>	<>	current:
DEP	Major Depressive Disorder	<>	<>	<>	past year:
DYS	Dysthymic Disorder	<>	<>	<>	
MAN	Mania	<>	<>	<>	
HYPOMAN	Hypomania	<>	<>	<>	
ENU	Enuresis	<>	<>	<>	
	Type: Nocturnal, Diurnal, Both				
ENC	Encopresis	<>	<>	<>	
SCZ	Schizophrenia	<>	<>	<>	
PSY	Psychosis	<>	<>	<>	

Psychosocial Stressors:

Other Stressors:

Behavioral Observations

Appearance: Affect:

Effort: Level of Activity:

Unusual Behaviors:

Presenting Problem

Home

1.

2.

School

1.

2.

3.

4.

5.

Peers/Work

1.

2.

3.

4.

5.

Medication

Type:

Dosage:

Child's Name: _____

Date: _____

ADHD	ODD	CD

A. Inattention
  1. \<a> \<b>
  2. \< >
  3. \<a> \<b>
  4. \<a> \<b> \<c>
  5. \< >
  6. \< >
  7. \< >
  8. \<a> \<b>
  9. \<a> \<b>
 	
B. Hyperactivity–Impulsivity
  1. \<a> \<b>
  2. \<a> \<b>
  3. \< >
  4. \<a> \<b>
  5. \< >
  6. \<a> \<b>
  7. \< >
  8. \<a> \<b>
  9. \<a> \<b> \<c>
	1. \<a> \<b>
	2. \<a> \<b>
	3. \<a> \<b> \<c> \<d>
	4. \< >
	5. \<a> \<b>
	6. \< >
	7. \< >
	8. \< >
		1. \< >
		2. \<a> \<b>
		3. \< >
		4. \< >
		5. \< >
		6. \< >
		7. \<a> \<b>
		8. \<a> \<b>
		9. \< >
		10. \<a> \<b>
		11. \< >
		12. \< >
		13. \< >
		14. \< >
		15. \<a> \<b>

Criteria If ≥6 in *A only*, then criteria met Inattentive \< > If ≥6 in *B only*, then criteria met Hyperactive–Impulsive \< > If ≥6 in A *and* ≥6 in B, then criteria met Combined \< >	**Criteria** If ≥4, then criteria met ODD \< >	**Criteria** If ≥3, then criteria met CD \< >

Duration
1. _____ (years old)
2. \< > _____ (years old)
3. \< > _____ (months)
 	
  * DUR met for ADHD \< >
	Duration
	1. _____ (years old)
	2. \< > _____ (years old)
	3. \< > _____ (months)
	
	  * DUR met for ODD \< >
		Duration
		1. _____ (years old)
		2. \< > _____ (years old)
		3. \< > _____ (months)
		
		  * DUR met for CD \< >

Impairment 1. \< > home 2. \< > school 3. \< > peers	**Impairment** 1. \< > home 2. \< > school 3. \< > peers	**Impairment** 1. \< > home 2. \< > school 3. \< > peers
		Type Childhood Onset \< > Adolescent Onset \< > Mild \< > Moderate \< > Severe \< >

SUB AB	PHO	SOCIAL PHO

1. < >
     <a>_____
     <b>_____
     <c>_____
 	
     _____
 2. < > _____
 3. < > _____
 4. < > _____
	1. _____
	   _____
	   _____
	 2. <a> <b>
	 3. <a> <b>
	 4. <ai> <aii> <aiii> <aiv> <b>
	 5. <a> <b>
		1. <a> <b>
		 2. < >
		 3. <a> <b>
		 4. <ai> <aii> <aiii> <aiv> <b>
		 5. < >

SUB AB	PHO	SOCIAL PHO

Duration
 1. _____ (years old)
 2. < > _____ (years old)
     _____ (months)
 	
    * DUR met for SUB AB < >
	Criteria
	   If 1–4, then criteria met
	       PHO < >
		Criteria
		   If 1–4, then criteria met
		     SOCIAL PHO < >

	Duration
	 1. _____ (years old)
	 2. < > _____ (years old)
	 3. < > _____ (months)
	
	    * DUR met for PHO < >
		Duration
		 1. _____ (years old)
		 2. < > _____ (years old)
		 3. < > _____ (months)
		
		   *DUR met for SOCIAL PHO < >

SUB AB	PHO	SOCIAL PHO
Impairment 1. <a> <b> 2. < > 3. <a> <b> 4. < >	**Impairment** 1. < > home 2. < > school 3. < > peers	**Impairment** 1. < > home 2. < > school 3. < > peers

Criteria
   If any use (Q1–4) and any
   impairment (1–4), then criteria
     met SUB AB < >
 	
 Type(s) _____
 _____
 _____
 _____
	Type(s)
	 Animal < >
	 Natural Environment < >
	 Blood–Injection–Injury < >
	 Situational < >
	 Other _____ < >	

SEP ANX	GEN ANX	OCD

1. <a> <b>
2. <a> <b>
3. < >
4. <a> <b>
5. <a> <b>
6. <a> <b>
7. <a> <b>
8. <a> <b>
	1. < > _____
	   _____
	   _____
	   _____
	   _____
	2. <a> <b>
	3. <a> <b> <c> <d> <e> <f>
		A. Compulsions
		   1. < > _____
		   2. <a> _____
		      <b>
		   3. < >
		
		B. Obsessions
		   1. <a> _____
		      <b> _____
		      <c> _____
		   2. <a> <b> <c>
		   3. < >
		
		C. Interference
		   1. <a> <b> <c>

Criteria If ≥3, then criteria met SEP ANX < >	**Criteria** If 1–3, then criteria met GEN ANX < >	**Criteria** If A1, A2, & C, then criteria met Compulsions < > If B1, B2, & C, then criteria met Obsessions < > If Compulsions + and/or Obsessions +, then criteria met OCD < >
Duration 1. _____ (years old) 2. < > _____ (years old) 3. < > _____ (weeks) *DUR met for SEP ANX < >	**Duration** 1. _____ (years old) 2. < > _____ (years old) 3. < > _____ (months) *DUR met for GEN ANX < >	**Duration** 1. _____ (years old) 2. < > _____ (years old) _____ (months) *DUR met for OCD < >
Impairment 1. < > home 2. < > school 3. < > peers	**Impairment** 1. < > home 2. < > school 3. < > peers	**Impairment** 1. < > home 2. < > school 3. < > peers

STRESS (ASD/PTSD)	ANO	BUL

A. Exposure
   1. \<a> \<b> _____
   2. \<a> \<b> \<c> \<d> \<e>
   3. \< > _____
B. Dissociation
   1. \<a> \<b> \<c> \<d>
   2. \< >
   3. \< >
   4. \< >
   5. \< >
C. Reexperiencing
   1. \<a> \<b> \<c>
   2. \<a> \<b>
   3. \<a> \<b>
   4. \<a> \<b>
   5. \< >
D. Avoidance
   1. \<a> \<b>
   2. \<a> \<b> \<c>
   3. \< >
   4. \<a> \<b>
   5. \<a> \<b>
   6. \<a> \<b>
   7. \<a> \<b>
E. Hyperarousal
   1. \<a> \<b>
   2. \<a> \<b>
   3. \< >
   4. \< >
   5. \< >
	1. \<a> \<b>
	2. \<a>
	   ht: _____
	   wt: _____
	  \<b>
	   ht: _____
	   wt: _____
	3. \<a> \<b> \<c>
	4. \<a> \<b> \<c>
	5. \< >
		1. \< > _____
		_____
		
		2. \<a> \<b> \<c> \<d>
		3. \<a> \<b> \<c> \<d>
		4. \<a> \<b>

Criteria If A1 *&* A2, ≥3 in B, ≥1 in C, ≥3 in D, and ≥2 in E, then criteria met ASD \< > If A1 *&* A2, ≥1 in C, ≥3 in D, and ≥2 in E, then criteria met PTSD \< >	**Criteria** If 1–4 (&5 for pubescent girls), then criteria met ANO \< >	**Criteria** If 1–4, then criteria met BUL \< >

Duration
1. _____ (years old)
2. \< > _____ (years old)
3. a. \< > _____ (weeks)
   b. \< >
   c. \< > _____ (days)
4. \< > _____ (months)
     *DUR met for ASD \< >
     *DUR met for PTSD \< >
	Duration
	1. _____ (years old)
	2. \< > _____ (years old)
	3. \< > _____ (months)
	
	    *DUR met for ANO \< >
		Duration
		1. _____ (years old)
		2. \< > _____ (years old)
		3. a. \< > _____ (#/week)
		   b. \< > _____ (months)
		
		    *DUR met for BUL \< >

Impairment 1. \< > home 2. \< > school 3. \< > peers	**Impairment** 1. \< > home 2. \< > school 3. \< > peers	**Impairment** 1. \< > home 2. \< > school 3. \< > peers
Type (PTSD) Acute \< > Regular Onset \< > Chronic \< > Delayed Onset \< >		

DEP/DYS (MDD/DD)	DEP/DYS (MDD/DD)	MAN/HYPOMAN

A. Dysphoric Mood
  1. \<a> \<b> \<c>
  2. \<a> \<bi> \<bii> \<biii>
    \<c> \<d>
 	
B. Loss of Interest
  1. \<a> \<b>
  2. \<a> \<b> \<c>
 	
C. Appetite Changes
  1. \<a> \<b> \<c>
  2. \<a> \<b>
 	
D. Sleep Changes
    Bedtime: _____
    Wakeup: _____
  1. \<a> \<b> \<c>
  2. \<a> \<b>
 	
E. Psychomotor Changes
  1. \<a> \<b> \<c> \<d>
  2. \<a> \<b>
 	
F. Low Energy
  1. \<a> \<b> \<c> \<d>
 	
G. Guilt
  1. \<a> \<b> \<c> \<d>
  2. \<a> \<b>
 	
H. Impaired Concentration
  1. \<a> \<b> \<c> \<d> \<e>
  2. \< >
 	
I. Hopelessness
  1. \<a> \<b> \<c>
 	
J. Morbid/Suicidal Thoughts
  1. \<a> \<b>
  2. \<a> \<b> \<c> \<d> \<e>
 	
_____
_____
_____
_____
_____
		A. Elevated Mood
		  1. \<a> _____
		    \<b> _____
		    \<c> _____
		  2. \< > _____
		
		B. Other Symptoms
		  1. \<a> _____
		    \<b>
		  2. \<a> \<b> \<c> _____
		  3. \<a> \<b> \<c> \<d>
		  4. \<a> \<b> \<c>
		  5. \< >
		  6. \<a> \<b> \<c> \<d> \<e>
		  7. \<a> \<b> \<c> \<d>
		
		C. Interference
		  1. \< >
		  2. \< >

	Criteria If A &/or B & ≥5 of A–H or J, then criteria met MDD \< > If A & ≥2 of C, D, F, G, H, or I, then criteria met DD \< >	**Criteria** If A1(a, b, & c) + ≥3 in B + ≥1 in C *or* A2 + ≥4 in B + ≥1 in C, then criteria met MAN \< > If A1(a, b, & c) + ≥3 in B + none in C *or* A2 + ≥4 in B + none in C, then criteria met HYPOMAN \< >

	Duration
	1. _____ (years old)
	2. \< > _____ (years old)
	3. MDD \< > _____ (weeks)
	   DD \< > _____ (months)
	
	  *DUR met for MDD \< >
	  *DUR met for DD \< >
		Duration
		1. _____ (years old)
		2. \< > _____ (years old)
		3. MAN \< > _____ (weeks)
		   HYPO \< > _____ (days)
		
		  *DUR met for MAN \< >
		  *DUR met for HYPOMAN \< >

	Impairment 1. \< > home 2. \< > school 3. \< > peers	**Impairment** 1. \< > home 2. \< > school 3. \< > peers

ENU	SCZ/PSY	STRESSORS

1. < >
 2. \<a> \<b>
 3. \<a> \<b>
	A. Psychotic Symptoms
	   1. \<a> \<b> \<c> \<d> \<e>
	   2. \<a> \<b> \<c> \<d> \<e> \<f>
	   3. < >
	   4. < >
	   5. < >
		A. Child Abuse/Neglect
		   1. \<a> \<b> \<c>
		   2. \<a> \<b> \<c> \<d>
		   3. \<a> \<b> \<c> \<d>
		   4. < >
		   5. < >

ENU

1. < >
2. \<a> \<b>
3. \<a> \<b>

Criteria

    If 1, ≥1 in 2, 3a, and 3b,
       then criteria met
          ENU < >

Duration

1. _____ (years old)
2. < > _____ (years old)
3. \<a> _____ (x/week)
   \<b> _____ (months)

   *DUR met for ENU < >

Impairment

1. < > home
2. < > school
3. < > peers

Type

Nocturnal   < >
Diurnal   < >
Both   < >

ENC

1. < >
2. < >

Criteria

If both 1 & 2, then criteria met
         ENC < >

Duration

1. _____ (years old)
2. < > _____ (years old)
3. \<a> _____ (x/month)
   \<b> _____ (months)

   *DUR met for ENC < >

Impairment

1. < > home
2. < > school
3. < > peers

SCZ/PSY

A. Psychotic Symptoms
  1. \<a> \<b> \<c> \<d> \<e>
  2. \<a> \<b> \<c> \<d> \<e> \<f>
  3. < >
  4. < >
  5. < >

B. Interference
  1. < >
  2. < >
  3. < >

Criteria

    If ≥2 in A and ≥1 in B,
      then criteria met
         SCZ < >

    If ≥1 in A, then criteria met
         PSY < >

Duration

1. _____ (years old)
2. < > _____ (years old)
3. < > _____ (months)

   *DUR met for SCZ < >
   *DUR met for PSY < >

Impairment

1. < > home
2. < > school
3. < > peers

STRESSORS

A. Child Abuse/Neglect
  1. \<a> \<b> \<c>
  2. \<a> \<b> \<c> \<d>
  3. \<a> \<b> \<c> \<d>
  4. < >
  5. < >

Duration

1. _____
2. < > _____
3. _____
4. _____
5. < >

B.   Other Stressors
  1.   \<a> \<b> \<c> \<d> \<e>
  2.   < >
  3.   \<a> \<b>
  4.   \<a> \<b> \<c>
  5.   \<a> \<b>
  6.   \<a> \<b>
  7.   \<a> _____
      \<b>
  8.   \<a> \<b> \<c> \<d>
  9.   < > _____
      _____
      _____
 10. < >
 11. < > _____
      _____
      _____